D1713460

The Myth
and Truth
About Ginseng

The Myth and Truth About Ginseng

JOSEPH P. HOU

South Brunswick and New York: A. S. Barnes and Company
London: Thomas Yoseloff Ltd.

A. S. Barnes and Co., Inc.
Cranbury, New Jersey 08512

Thomas Yoseloff Ltd
Magdalen House
136-148 Tooley Street
London SE1 2TT, England

Library of Congress Cataloging in Publication Data

Hou, Joseph P., 1929-
   The myth and truth about ginseng.

   Includes bibliographical references and index.
   1. Ginseng — Therapeutic use.   2. Ginseng.
3. Medicine, Chinese.   I. Title
RS165.G45H68   615'.323'48   77-74114
ISBN 0-498-02083-5

PRINTED IN THE UNITED STATES OF AMERICA

CONTENTS

FOREWORD

In the past few years, increasing contacts between the United States and the People's Republic of China have brought to the fore various aspects of traditional Chinese science and medicine. A very important aspect as noted by Western observers is the combining of observations or experiences accumulated during thousands of years of Chinese culture and the very latest scientific and medical knowledge of the Western world. One notable example of this combination has been the recent success of Chinese scientists in predicting earthquakes. Various natural and unusual phenomena associated with earthquakes have been combined with Western geophysical sciences to effectively foretell the occurrence of an earthquake. Without doubt, this Chinese achievement is equally valuable to other countries in the world to reduce the horrendous toll on human life and industry.

Increasingly, various aspects of Chinese medicine are becoming known to the West. Both acupuncture therapy, an ancient Chinese healing art, and acupuncture anesthesia, a modern Chinese development, have received a great deal of notoriety in the last few years. However, the lack of knowledge about these subjects has led to a great deal of misunderstanding of the uses of these medical techniques.

So it is with Chinese herbal medicine. A recent experience detailed in a well-known medical journal described the reluctance of American doctors to have therapy recommended by an eminent Chinese cardiologist instituted for an American who had had a myocardial infarction while on a visit to China because they were unfamiliar with one of the herbal remedies recommended. In the treatment of diseases, the application of herbals in Chinese medicine is not totally unfounded. For example, acute appendicitis has been treated successfully with herbal remedies without surgery. Mechanistically, the anti-appendicitis drugs can effectively promote peristalsis in addition to blood flow to the appendix, thus the bacteria and the toxic materials can promptly be eliminated from the lumen of the appendix. Only in the last few years have herbal preparations somewhat familiar to Westerners, such as ginseng, been the subject of much discussion, some of it fact and some of it fable. Needless to say, ginseng has been in use for thousands of years and the observations of its effects are numerous. These observations are now becoming the subject of Western scientific scrutiny.

The Myth and Truth About Ginseng relates the fabulous history of ginseng. It also encompasses the latest scientific observations of some of the chemical, pharmacological, and clinical aspects of ginseng. It is hoped that this volume will give Western scientists and physicians an insight into the uses and effects of ginseng and spur their interests to investigate further the pharmacological and biomedical effects ascribed to it. Hopefully, it will also interest the scientific and medical world in other entities used in traditional Chinese medicine in the treatment and prevention of diseases.

C. P. Li, M.D.
Former Chief
Virus Biology Section
L.V.R., D.B.S.
National Institute of Health
Bethesda
President, The American
Center for Chinese Medicine

PREFACE

The prime aim of this book is to provide new evidence from scientific studies of ginseng, thus answering the questions most frequently asked:

1. Does ginseng really work?
2. Does ginseng prevent fatigue? If so, is it useful for athletics?
3. Is ginseng useful for combating stress?
4. Is ginseng an aphrodisiac agent?
5. Is ginseng useful for controlling diabetes and hypertension?
6. How can I grow my own ginseng plant?
7. How can ginseng help me achieve rejuvenation and longevity?
8. Where can I buy ginseng and how much does it cost?

In the early spring of 1976, about nine thousand chemists, chemical engineers, scientists, and delegates from more than one hundred foreign and domestic scientific organizations gathered in New York City to celebrate the hundredth anniversary of the founding of the American Chemical Society.* In the ceremonial session of the centennial meeting on Monday, April 5th, the world-famous scientist and Nobel laureate Linus Lauling addressed the audience, saying:

> I believe that the goal that we should strive to reach during the third century of the United States of America is that of constructing a country in which every person has the possibility of leading a good life.

In trying to achieve this objective, "the principle of the minimization of suffering" should be applied. Dr. Pauling further emphasized how to minimize human suffering while maximizing happiness and pursuing longevity:

*Chemical Engineering News (April 19, 1976), pp. 33-36.

9

physicians have observed that the death of a person at an early age usually is accompanied by a rather large amount of suffering, whereas that of a very old person, 90 or 100 years old, is not accompanied, on the average, by so much suffering. There accordingly would be value to discovering how to increase the life expectancy and slow down the process of aging, and, of course, to decrease the mortality from cancer and other diseases that might be described as causing death to occur in an inhumane manner. During the coming century chemists and other investigators will, I believe, succeed in finding the regimes, nutritional and environmental, that would lead in a *decreased rate of aging* and *increased life expectancy.* . . .

As a matter of fact, what Dr. Pauling has in mind—the agent that we desire to minimize suffering and to increase the life expectancy—may be already available on earth, but we Americans, including the distinguished physical chemist Dr. Pauling, fail to recognize its existence. It is the so-called manroot, ginseng.

For more than forty centuries the Chinese, as well as other Asians, have continuously praised the exotic ginseng root for the healing power they believe it to possess. In at least forty diseases, including nervous and gastrointestinal disorders, all forms of debility, hypertension, diabetes, and diseases of the heart, liver, and kidney found in the classical Chinese *materia medica* books (*pen-ts'ao*), ginseng may prove to be effective. Yet what ginseng could assist you to achieve or maintain in strength, vitality, rejuvenation, and longevity, sounds more attractive to the majority of the people, particularly the aging. There must be medicinal qualities, otherwise ginseng would not have been called "divine herb," "immortal herb," and "herb of the spirit" in the Orient and sold at prices ten to one hundred times higher than silver or gold of its own weight by the Chinese druggists in the old days.

To Western doctors, traditional Chinese herbal medicine is somewhat irrational, enigmatic, and at best, empirical and nonscientific. The herb drugs are nothing but primitive remedies with a lack of predictable efficacy. However, there are many open-minded Western scientists and medical doctors who have quite different opinions, and most important of all, who do not think Chinese medicine is unfounded or based on superstition.

Professors Takagi, Watanabe, and Ishii of the University of Tokyo, said recently:*

No pharmacologically violent principles are found in prescriptions of Oriental [Chinese] medicine. Their main ingredients exert so mild an activity that they cannot change normal conditions of living organisms, but rather exhibit a normalizing effect on abnormal conditions of the patient. In Oriental medicine, the use of a single medicine is very rare, various ingredients contained in one prescription present a synergistic or antagonistic effect according to the physical conditions of the patient. The isolated principle from the plant may not represent the entire therapeutic effect of the whole plant.

In view of the vast differences in the cultural backgrounds and medical systems of the Soviet Union and China, it is hard to perceive the profound interest of the Russian scientists in Chinese medicinal herbs, particularly ginseng. The distinguished pharmacologist and physician Professor I. I. Brekhman and his associates of the Academy of Sciences, Vladivostok, USSR, have spent more than twenty five years in ginseng research. Dr. Brekhman has written:

Medical science has not yet studied even a small part of the consolidated experience gained by the Chinese in the course of time. Oriental [Chinese] medicine dealt primarily with natural products rather than with synthetic ones. . . . Oriental medicine employs drugs of low toxicity. The drugs do not produce a quick symptomatic effect, but rather work slowly and very often efficaciously to increase natural resistance and recuperative power of the patient.

Professor Brekhman also said that ginseng is one of the most interesting traditional remedies that merits serious study.**

Since World War II, ginseng has become an increasingly important plant, receiving considerable recent publicity in the press all over the world. As a result, significant changes have taken place. One of the changes is that ginseng has become the

---

*Chen, K. K. and B. Mukerji, eds., *Pharmacology of Oriental Plants*, Pergamon Press, New York, 1965, p. 1.

**Brekhman, I. I. and I. V. Drdymov, *Lloyda*, *32*: 46-51 (1969).

subject of intensive chemical and biological research in China, Japan, Korea, Bulgaria, the Soviet Union, and more recently, parts of Western Europe. One of the most noteworthy endeavors of ginseng research is to give the benefits of its achievements to ever wider circles of the world's population. Another notable change is the increase in ginseng cultivation centers in China, Japan, the USSR, and Korea, and the building up of quite a number of modern and collective ginseng farms for industrialized production to meet the ever-increasing international demands for ginseng tonic products and, most important of all, to lower the price.

Natural products remain the primary source of supply of many clinically useful drugs of ancient heritage. For example, at the discovery of salicin in the bark of willow trees, no one could predict that one day it could be developed as the most remarkable, most versatile, and most widely prescribed drug in history — aspirin. For centuries, the natives of India chewed snakeroot (*Rauwolfia cerpentina*) for its calming effect. Soon after the isolation of reserpine from the snakeroot it became an exceedingly important tranquilizer and an agent in the treatment and control of hypertension. With the discovery of Mexican yams, an abundant, inexpensive source or raw material for the synthesis of numerous steroid hormones became available. Ephedra, ergot, opium, digitalis, and penicillin are other examples of many natural agents that have become contemporary therapeutic remedies. The real beauty of natural products is their low incidence of toxicity, which we desire.

Today, in the search for new therapeutic agents (synthetic chemicals, of course), the Western pharmaceutical industries usually examine hundreds and thousands of potential candidates of which only a few are clinically investigated. A very small number or none of these candidates ultimately reach the marketplace. Drug companies spend an average of five to ten years and more than $12,000,000 to develop one new drug. Even so, they still *cannot* guarantee its complete safety.

Ginseng is an age-old medicine, and its value in promoting health and happiness has long been recognized in the Orient. Yet it is a rather new wonder substance to Western people. Many people in the Western countries, particularly young

Americans, have discovered ginseng only recently, and many of them are still wondering what ginseng is. This is because ginseng is not popular at all in the United States. Also, a literature gap exists between the East and West on ginseng. Although many legendary stories and tales about ginseng now prevail in books on herbs and medicinal plants, they are written fictitiously and erroneously to make ginseng appear more attractive and curious to the reader. None of these legends is scientific or factual. The modern scientific evidence on the pharmacological properties and the potential clinical usefulness of ginseng published in the Orient and in the Soviet Union is totally lacking in virtually all American libraries.

As a China-born American pharmaceutical chemist and senior scientist, I have been studying ginseng for more than thirty years, and I am also a ginseng enthusiast and user. From my own experience and from that of several members in my family, indeed, ginseng works. For it kept me disease free, young looking, and most important of all, able to utilize my time more efficiently and more productively to accomplish whatever I wanted to do. The relatively healthy and long lives of many members of my family confirms the longevity effect of ginseng. From my past thirty years of experience, it has been proven to me that ginseng is valuable in my life, and I wish its benefits to be extended to the reader as well. This book is written with this purpose.

This book is made up of twelve chapters separated into three parts. The philosophical and technical features of traditional Chinese medicine are introduced in chapter 1. The concept of Chinese medicine is little heard by the American public and it is essential to the understanding of the use of ginseng and other herbal medicine in the Oriental [Chinese] medical practice.

Chapter 2 tells what ginseng is, the history of *Panax ginseng* in China, and its virtues in Chinese medicine.

The ginseng plants found in Korea, Japan, Siberia, and the Himalayas are covered in chapters 3 and 4.

Chapter 5 is devoted to *Panax quinquefolium* — American ginseng — and the history of its discovery in North America.

To the business-minded readers, chapter 6 will be of interest. It tells of the trade of American ginseng in the Chinese market in the past, the story of ginseng hunting, and the current flourishing ginseng business in Korea and Japan. A list of ginseng dealers is also provided.

If you are interested in growing your own ginseng plant you must read chapter 7 carefully. It provides all the information necessary to grow ginseng.

As a result of the information gap on ginseng between the East and the West, the majority of the population in the United States knows little about the latest development on ginseng. You will find this in chapter 8.

Chapter 9 focuses on the chemistry of *panax ginseng* — the active constituents contained in *P. ginseng* and other ginseng species found in Asia, America, and Siberia.

This scientific evidence: how ginseng really works, what it can do for you, and can ginseng make old people young is summarized in chapters 10, 11 and 12. The results of biological (animal) and clinical (human) studies on ginseng by hundreds of scientists all over the world in the past fifty years are covered in these three chapters.

This compendium covers a wide range of information about ginseng: from the manroot story to ginseng hunting, from the two-man walk test to the inhibition of amnion cell aging, and from panaquilon to ginsenoside. This presentation of information moves from the myths to the truths about ginseng. This is the first book in the English language that has ever attempted to encompass the currently available material about the little-known manroot.

A Glossary, which contains the most important and commonly encountered scientific (chemical, pharmacological, and medical) terms used in this book, is also provided.

It should be noted that I make no medical or therapeutic claims for any of the herbal remedies including ginseng listed in this book although these herbal remedies have been used for thousands of years in the Orient and are reported safe. Like any medicine, these materials should be used with care and should be discussed with physicians who know herbal medicine.

Finally, I wish to express my gratitude to the library of Squibb Institute for Medical Research, National Library of

Medicine, Gest Oriental Library of Princeton University, The Office of Monoploy, Korea, and Pharmaton Limited, Lugano, Switzerland, for providing valuable references and information on ginseng research. I am also grateful to Mrs. M. Cardona for her valuable assistance in preparing the Glossary of this book.

The Myth
and Truth
About Ginseng

Superior numbers in the text correspond to references that follow chapter 12.

PART I

The Mysterious Elixir of Life: Ginseng

1
THE CHINESE STYLE
OF HEALING AND
HERBAL MEDICINE

TRADITIONAL CHINESE MEDICINE

Traditional Chinese medicine, or *Chung-I*, is the daily medical practice in China. *Chung-I* incorporates traditional techniques and methods as well as herbal medicine.

The medicinal agents used for healing are primarily natural products rather than synthetic chemicals. These natural products are derived not only from herbaceous and arboreous species, but also from animal and mineral sources. The Chinese physician tailors his treatment to fit the individual patient's condition as well as the nature of the disease. His prescriptions usually contain many medicinal substances to produce synergistic action, or to neutralize negative interactions, and to mask the bitter taste of the crude drugs. These drugs are administered, in most cases, in the form of a decoction.[1,2] Chinese medicine recognizes complex mixtures of drugs, and does not appreciate the advantage or effectiveness of a single drug entity. This is a fundamental difference between Chinese and Western medicine.

Acupuncture, the insertion of slender solid needles into specific points in the body, is a rather elaborate technique of *Chung-I*. Acupuncture therapy has also been used in Korea, Japan, and other Southeast Asian countries for thousands of years, and in France for more than a century. A small but

21

growing group of British physicians use acupuncture. It is practiced in Germany, and as long as their love affair with China endured, the Russians used acupuncture and conducted extensive research on acupuncture. And finally, the people of Canada and of the United States suddenly, and with characteristic fervor, have discovered acupuncture.[3] Acupuncture analgesia, a highly sophisticated medical technique developed in China only fifteen years ago, has been more impressive and convincing than therapeutic acupuncture. In China it has now been accepted and is used in surgery in nearly all general hospitals.[4]

In the last few years, the term *acupuncture* has become familiar in the United States. The question raised in 1962 about its usefulness has been answered by a great number of American doctors who have seen it applied in the People's Republic of China. Most of these Western observers have been astounded by the extraordinary effect of the acupuncture needles in producing surgical anesthesia, profound enough for the performance of surgical operations.

The New York Times correspondent James Reston experienced acupuncture therapy in a Peking general hospital. The journalist, as well as all other American physicians who subsequently visited China, observed and testified to the fact that acupuncture was "verity" and "no delusion." They brought back from the People's Republic of China irrefutable proof in the form of films depicting the performance of major surgery under acupuncture analgesia with immediate and complete postsurgical functioning of the patient.[5]

Although surgery has not been as widely applied as acupuncture therapy in traditional Chinese medicine, some special surgical techniques do exist. A method of cataract surgery called "coughing," with a site of scleral incision, had been used centuries ago in China.[4]

In addition to herbal medicine, acupuncture, and surgery, physical therapy, diet therapy, and massage are other features and techniques of traditional *Chung-I*. Massage was fully developed during the T'ang dynasty. The simpler hand movements of massage supposedly stimulate circulation and make muscles and joints supple, thus reducing pain. The diet therapy is even less known to Westerners, although it is an indispensable part of Chinese medicine. The first compendium on diet therapy, written by Sung Ssu-Miao, was published in the T'ang dynasty; several other related books on diet therapy were also published during the late T'ang and Sung dynasties. These books discuss the properties, uses, and amounts of specific food substances for diet therapy and prevention of diseases.

Practitioners of *Chung-I* are generally divided into herbalist and acupuncturist groups. The former turn to an enormous *materia medica* based on the pharmacological properties of herbal remedies. Ginseng (*Panax ginseng*) is the most popular drug and has been prescribed in practically every prescription—for weakness, debility, fever, chills, cough, pallor, and, of course, to enhance virility and restore health. However, the majority of people cannot afford to pay the extravagant price for ginseng. So Chinese doctors often prescribe substitute substances: American ginseng, Japanese ginseng, or other wonder roots such as Hsuan-shen, Kú-shen, Sha-shen, Tzu-shen, and Tang-shen instead of genuine ginseng.

The practice of traditional medicine is followed not only in China, but also in Japan, Korea, Taiwan, Indochina, Singapore, and other parts of Southeast Asia, and by at least eighteen million overseas Chinese. Thus, a third of the world's people (the Orientals) receive some form of traditional Chinese medicine. For this reason, the term *Oriental medicine* has been used by Westerners to describe the traditional medical practice in the Orient.

In Chinese history, [6,7] the three legendary emperors Fu-Hsi, Shen-Nung, and Huang-Ti are the founders of early Chinese civilization. To Fu-Hsi is attributed the *Canon of Changes* or *I-Ching*, regarded as the most ancient Chinese philosophy and medicine. Shen-Nung, also known as Yin-Ti, is the father of agriculture and herbal medicine. It is said that he tasted hundreds of herbs and other crude drugs in order to acquaint himself with their properties and usefulness. He is commonly attributed the compilation of the first *Pen-ts'ao*, or Chinese *materia medica*. Huang-Ti, the Yellow Emperor, contributed a complete treatise on the principles of health and medicine in

2697 B.C., known as *Huang Ti Nei Ching Su-Wen (The Yellow Emperor's Classic of Internal Medicine)* or simply called *Nei Ching (The Canon of Medicine)*, which consisted of eighteen volumes with 162 chapters.[7] Although it was written more than four thousand years ago, it has been recognized as a most valuable treatise on internal medicine and supposedly the world's oldest extant medical book. Traditional Chinese medicine can claim to be the world's first organized body of medical knowledge.[8]

The Canon of Medicine was also the most interesting medical book that ever existed. It was compiled in the form of a dialogue between the emperor and his physician minister, Ch'i-Pai.[7] Their discussions ranged over the philosophy of nature, theories of yin-yang, The Five Elements doctrine, pulse diagnosis, mechanisms of viscera, vascular systems, the value of life, and the achievement of the perfect body. The same book also illustrated that the prevention of disease can be achieved by regular habits, proper diet, a suitable combination of work and rest, and the maintenance of peaceful mind.

EARLY MEDICAL PHILOSOPHY

Traditional Chinese medicine is also the most pervasive and the most unyielding of the indigenous systems. It is based on the tenet that a human being is a microcosm constantly interacting with the immense universe, which influences and also controls every aspect of his life, including his health.[3]

As a matter of fact, early Chinese medicine incorporated philosophy and religion. Three essential religious philosophy concepts that control early medical thinking are *Tao, yin-yang theory*, and the *Doctrine of Five Elements.*[7]

Tao. During the sixth century B.C., Lao Tzu, the spiritual father of Taoism, founded the natural philosophy. Taoism is a concept common to all Chinese. It is the key to the mysterious intermingling of Heaven and Earth. Tao means "Way" and the method of maintaining the harmony between this world and the beyond. As in an agricultural society, the ancient Chinese philosophy is always related to nature and cosmology. The only manner in which man could attain the right Tao was by emulating the course of the universe and adjusting completely to it.

Tao plays an important role as the regulator of the universe and the highest code of conduct. A man's health and longevity depend highly on his behavior toward Tao. Longevity itself became to a certain degree a token of sainthood, since it was an indication that it had been achieved by personal effort of complete adherance to Tao. Those who follow Tao achieve the formula of perpetual youth and maintain a youthful body.

Yin and Yang Theory. Yin and yang are the shady side of a hill (yin) and the sunny side of a hill (yang) from literary translation. Yang stands for sun, heaven, day, fire, heat, dryness, light, and many other positive and masculine subjects, while yin represents moon, earth, night, water, cold, damp, dark, and many negative and feminine subjects. Yang means motion, hence life; yin means standstill, hence death. The principle of yin and yang is the basis of the entire universe. It is the principle of everything in creation. However, it must be borne in mind that yin and yang are conceived as one entity and that both together are ever present. Day changes into night, spring and summer change to autumn and winter, light changes into dark, etc. From these striking manifestations it was deduced that all happenings in nature as well as in human life were conditions caused by the constantly changing relationship of yin and yang.

Heat is yang and cold is yin. In the human body excessive yang causes fever, and excessive yin causes chills. Every food or medicament has a predominant character, either of yin or yang. The art of healing is to ascertain where and in which direction the equipoise of yin or yang has been lost the balance, then the appropriate medication or treatment has to be applied to restore it to normal, and to restore the internal balance and harmony. This is the essence of Chinese medical thinking.

The *Nei Ching* provides us with many examples of this interchange between yin and yang and of the duality preserved within a single thing. As to the interrelation of yin and yang in man, male belongs to yang, female belongs to yin, yet both male and female are products of the two elements, hence both qualities are contained in both sexes. In the dual nature of yin and yang within the human body, yin and yang correspond to the surface and the interior, respectively. The yin and yang in harmony means health; disharmony or undue preponderance of one element brings disease and death. Man received the doctrine of Tao as a means of maintaining perfect balance and securing for himself health and long life.[7]

The Doctrine of Five Elements More tangible components of yin and yang are the five elements. Yin and yang, in addition to exerting dual existence, are subdivided into metal, wood, water, fire, and earth—the so-called five elements. Man was said to be the product of heaven and earth by the interaction of yin and yang, and therefore contains the five elements.

The sequence of the five elements varies according to the viewpoint from which they are enumerated. The *Nei Ching* explains the mutual victories of the five elements as follows:

Wood brought in contact with metal is felled;
fire brought in contact with water is extinguished;
earth brought in contact with wood is penetrated;
metal brought in contact with fire is dissolved;
water brought in contact with earth is halted.

The sequence of subjugations is that metal subjugates wood; water subjugates fire; wood subjugates earth; fire subjugates metal; and earth subjugates water.

The doctrine of Five Elements also extends to grains, fruits, animals, vegetables, flavors, odors, climates, musical notes, human organs, and many groups, each of which contains five components. The five grains that act as nourishment are wheat, glutinous millet, millet, rice and beans. The five fruits are peaches, plums, apricots, chestnuts, and dates. The five domestic animals that contribute additional nutrients are fowl, sheep, beef, horses, and pigs. The five vegetables are mallows, coarse greens, scallions, onions, and leeks. The human body contains five viscera: liver, lungs, heart, spleen, and kidneys.

The *Nei Ching* gives the following explanations of how the natural elements affect the human body. The climate elements affect the viscera of our body; heat injures the heart; cold injures the lungs; wind injures the liver; humidity injures the spleen; and dryness injures the kidney.

The five viscera, of course, control the body. The heart controls the pulse; the lungs control the skin; the liver controls the muscles; the spleen controls the flesh; and the kidney controls the bones. The five spiritual resources of our body are also controlled by the five viscera. The liver controls the soul; the heart controls the spirit; the spleen controls ideas; the lungs conrol the animal spirit (ghost); the kidney controls the will.

The five flavors affect the body in the following manner: salty flavor hardens the pulse; bitter flavor withers the skin; pungent flavor knots the muscles; sour flavor toughens the flesh; and sweet flavor causes aches in the bones. The five flavors are said to be effective not only upon the five viscera but also upon all parts of the body that are connected with the five viscera. If people pay attention to the five flavors and blend them well, their bones will remain straight, their muscles will remain tender and young, breath and blood will circulate freely, the pores will be fine in texture, and consequently breath and bones will be filled with the essence of life.[7]

THE FEATURES AND TECHNIQUES
OF CHINESE MEDICINE

Diagnosis Diagnosis in Chinese medicine, or *zue-chen,* is listed in *Nei Ching.* There are four basic methods of diagnosis of the patient. They are: visual observation, questioning about case history, auditory systems, and taking the pulse. Chinese *pulsology,* developed in a great detail by Wang Shu-ho, recognizes three spots along the radial artery of each wrist, detected with the tips of three fingers. The pulse readings reflect the functioning of different viscera. In Chinese medicine, pulse-taking has been the chief method of diagnosis. At the three pulse spots each wrist has a deep and a superficial reading, thus giving a total of twelve different pulses in all. If the patient is a female, the right radial artery is palpated first; if a male, the left. The rate, strength, and direction of the beat in each segment of the pulse are determined. A strong pulse indicates a yang-type disease, while a weak pulse represents a yin-type disease. Only experienced doctors can diagnose malfunction of any part of the internal organs. Obviously this is quite a different diagnosis technique from that in Western medicine. The art of pulse diagnosis is extremely complex in the way it works. This has been the chief point of controversy between those who understand and those who do not.

Acupuncture Acupuncture is another important branch of Chinese medicine. The therapeutic art of acupuncture (not acupuncture anesthesia) had been fully developed by the time of *Nei Ching*, in which an elaborate description of the practice and principles were recorded.

The rationale of acupuncture historically has been based on stimulation of a *Ching-lo* system. *Ching-lo* is a system of channels and ducts that is anatomically distinct from the circulatory or nervous systems. Acupuncture has been used to cure many diseases. It is used most spectacularly to alleviate deafness and induce anesthesia. A publication from the Research Institute in Peking makes the following grandiose claims:

> Preliminary observations show that acupuncture...can exert influence on the visible elements of the blood, the peristalsis and secretion of the stomach and intestines, and the secretion of bile; stimulate the kidney's power of excretion, and improve the conditions of blood pressure and cardiac impulse, increase the amount of immunizing agents in the body, and stimulate cytocannibalism. . . produce curative effects of the central nervous system, segmental reflex, blood, and local parts of the body.[3]

In the classical system of Chinese medicine acupuncture is used in both diagnosis and treatment. The theoretical basis is the system of acupuncture points distributed along the meridian, each linked with one or more internal organs. At least 361 acupuncture points have been identified. The fundamental concept of acupuncture is that detailed knowledge of the distribution of these points allows both diagnosis and treatment. Malfunction of an organ may be recognized by hypersensitivity of the corresponding acupuncture points, and relieved by stimulation at the irritable point. In general, arthritis, neuritis, and paralysis after nerve injury or stroke are among the disorders treated most successfully. In these conditions the needles are stimulated electrically, usually with a square-wave alternating pulse at about two hundred cycles per minute. The power source is a six-volt battery. This stimulation causes obvious muscular twitching at the site of insertion of the needle but apparently no great discomfort for the patient. Acupuncture therapy has also been widely used in the treatment of angina, to relieve cardiac pain, for analgesic effect in childbirth, in migraine, and in many chronic skeletal disorders.[8]

Anesthesia with acupunture has been so successful that it has been regarded as the most bizarre branch of Chinese medicine by Western doctors. Actually acupuncture for anesthesia is a new technique in Chinese medicine. It has been successfully applied in operations on the thyroid, the eye, the heart, the brain, and in hernia repair. Thyroid operations, for example, seem to be done under acupuncture frequently. The procedure has apparently been much simplified in recent years: at one time up to thirty needles might be used to achieve anesthesia, but now it is commonplace for only two to be used. Both electrical stimulation and manual rotation of the needles were equally successful. Acupuncture is used far less for abdominal surgery and seems to be used very little for emergency operations or for the treatment of fractures. In the last few years, taking the whole range of surgery done in major hospitals, about ten to fifteen percent of the operations were conducted under acupuncture anesthesia. This is because, according to Chinese experts, it is difficult to achieve adequate muscular relaxation for abdominal surgery, and manipulation of internal viscera by the surgeon can cause the patient to experience unpleasant sensations. These apparently are the drawbacks of acupuncture anesthesia applied in China to date.[8]

China's Hsin-hwa News Agency recently reported that acupuncture anesthesia was successful in ninety-five percent of the trials on 360 horses and other animals. The fact that so many horses, mules, donkeys, cattle, and pigs have responded to the method should be an eloquent denial of some skeptics' visioning that success with human beings has been due to psychological preparation (Hsin-hwa News Agency, November 20, 1972). Other reports from the veterinary medicine field state that acupuncture will increase milk production in cows and the speed of racing horses.[3]

External Medication As to external medication, certain manipulative arts, notable massage, reduction of dislocation, treatment of fractures, and bone setting have been carried out with a high degree of practical skill. The traditional methods of treating fractures are very different from those in the West. In the traditional way, reduction of the fracture is achieved slowly, using short splint fixed with bandages over soft paper or cloth padding. The splints maintain alignment of the fracture but they are not designed to immobilize the joints above and below it. The rationale of the treatment is that the muscles and joints around the fracture should retain their mobility; exercise is encouraged, and the splints are adjusted as often as necessary to cope with the progressive reduction in the swelling around the injury. It is said that in simple fractures for which it is best used, traditional treatment achieves rapid relief of pain and swelling and allows early mobilization; the fractures heal more quickly than those treated in plaster, and the functional results are better.[8]

Cupping and Moxibustion These are less well-known techniques to Western physicians; both are age-old medical techniques in the treatment of counterirritation. Cupping is used for conditions such as backache, in which the mouth of a metal cup is heated and then applied to the selected area of the skin. Cooling of the air inside the cup forms a partial vacuum so causing suction and the formation of a hematoma. Moxibustion is another technique occasionally used in traditional Chinese medicine. The treatment is conducted in conjunction with acupuncture. After insertion of the acupuncture needles into the afflicted area of the body, a ball of moxa is applied to the outer end of the needle and ignited. The moxa ball burns for a few minutes, emitting a fair amount of both heat and smoke. Good results have been obtained in patients with frozen shoulder, sciatica, and musculoskeletal disorders.[8]

THE CHINESE HERBAL REMEDIES

The Chinese consistently refer to their herbal remedies as being the product of four thousand years of the people's struggle against disease, and cite the millennial endurance of these remedies as adequate empirical proof of their effectiveness. The raw materials of traditional herbal remedies include not only more than one thousand five hundred plants — dry leaves, barks, fruits, roots, stems, flowers, seeds, and nuts — but also such exotic objects as snakes, newts, stalactites, agates, and antlers. These remedies are either given as teas, decoctions, infusions, or as a mixture compounded from the raw materials after processing by much the same techniques as those used by herbalists in the West, i.e., drying, shredding, grinding, boiling, or infusing with certain solvents to extract the active principles. More than ten types of pharmaceutical preparations, such as powders, granules, pills, masses (in the form of a golfball), solutions, tinctures, medicated dressings, adhesive plasters, ointments, and pastes, are commonly found in the classical Chinese drugstores. Usually, the granules, pills, and masses are coated with preservatives or stores in beeswaxed shells to preserve the drug from oxidation and moisture decomposition.

Evolution of Herbal Medicine It is believed that in ancient times, while fighting for survival, the Chinese and people in other parts of the world must have acquired experience in selecting naturally available materials and to concoct healing potions to eliminate pain, reduce fever, control suffering, counteract diseases, and heal wounds. By trial and error, they gained practical knowledge that was useful in determining what minerals, or animals, and which parts of specific plants possess the desired healing activities and which ought to be discarded because of their toxicity. Knowledge concerning their medicinal properties and instructions as to their correct uses have been handed down from one generation to the next. In the course of time, a substantial volume of information of herbal remedies was thus accumulated. These crude drugs were classified and compiled in a compendium known as herbal or *materia medica*, and the particular name of *Pen-ts'ao* is used in Chinese medicine.

In Western civilization, Hippocrates (460-370B.C.) has been referred to as the Father of Western Medicine.[9,10] Dioscorides wrote his *De Materia Medica* in A.D. 78. In it, he described six hundred plants that were known to have healing power. Galen (A.D. 131-201) was most famous for his experience in herbal medicines and his pharmaceutical preparations. Yet it was more than five hundred years ahead of Galen that the Chinese *Pen-ts'ao* had been fully developed and systematized.

Numerous valuable drugs were derived from nature not only in China but in other parts of the world as well. Morphine, digitalis, quinine, atropine, ephedrine, and reserpine are examples of outstanding remedies developed from herbal medicine.

In the People's Republic of China most of the herbs grew wild in the past. Herbs are grown on state or national farms today. The people have been encouraged to exploit the mountainous areas that are most suitable for cultivation of herbs. Provinces in South China (Kwang-tung, Kwang-si, Yun-nan, Kwei-chow, and Sze-chwan) are the leading medicinal herb producing regions. The experimental plantation of the Institute of Materia Medica located in the western outskirt of Peking is one of the biggest government-controlled medicinal herb cultivation centers. About one thousand five hundred species of herbs are under cultivation in an area of about sixty-four acres. In the past years, about ten thousand barefoot doctors have been trained there each year to be thoroughly familiar with the commonly used herbal remedies. The experimental station maintains cultivated ginseng plants with special attention to sunlight and diseases.

PEN-TS'AO

Perhaps China is the richest country in the world in natural medicine. These medicinal agents have been studied by scholars and physicians in the past forty decades, classified, and recorded systematically in the compendia called *Pen-ts'ao*.

for different diseases. Dr. Hwa excelled as a surgeon in the palace and was the first surgeon to apply general anesthesia, which he produced by means of an unknown drug dissolved in wine.

After a long period of civil war and foreign tribes' invasion (about four hundred years) came the famous and most prosperous T'ang dynasty in Chinese history. In addition to the well-founded government system and social orders, a new medical service was also established. The Ministry of General Medical Service was set up in A.D. 624 to govern medical affairs as well as to examine the medical practitioners. The first medical college and hospital were also formed in the capitol of Ch'ang-an. Emperor Kao Tsung (reigned 650-683) ordered Li, Hsun, and Su, Ching, to organize a task force of twenty-two scholars and physicians to review the traditional *Pen-ts'ao*. After a few years of hard work, *Hsin-hsiu Pen-ts'ao* was published officially in A.D. 659 as the official pharmacopoeia of China. This book illustrates in detail the old and 114 new medicaments in twenty-five volumes. The medical advancement of China soon spread to other Asian countries. Without delay Korean (three kingdoms) and later Japanese governments were sending envoys, professionals, and students to China for studies.

In addition to medical achievements, foreign trade, culture, and religion were also flourishing during the T'ang dynasty. A very well-educated scholar and physician, Dr. Sung, Ssu-miao (581-682), after years of laborous studies of medicine and the religious doctrines of Taoism, Confucianism, Canon of Chung Tze, and Buddhism, he finally became a Buddhist Monk physician and lived as a hermit. He was summoned by two emperors, Wen Ti and Kao Tsung, who offered him a high position in the government, but he refused them all and returned to live to his hermitage. For the rest of his life he practiced as a physician and edited many books, both medical and religious. The most famous medical books he published were *Chien Chin Yao fung* and *Chien chin I fung (the Thousand Ducat Prescriptions* and the *Supplement to the Thousand Ducat Prescriptions)*. The remedies for the treatment of diseases of women, children, tumors, and intoxicated and oph-

The *Pen-ts'ao* in Chinese medicine is actually a combination of *materia medica*, pharmacology, and pharmacopoeia. Although Shen-nung is commonly attributed the editing of the first *Pen-ts'ao*, it was not until the Late Han dynasty that the great work of *Shen-nung Pen-ts'ao Ching* was formally published as the first official dispensatory (pharmacopoeia) in Chinese history. It contains 365 different medicaments, 237 from botanical, 65 from animal, 43 from mineral sources, and 20 of unknown origin. According to their properties and usefulness, these medicaments were classified into superior (first), middle (second), and inferior (third) classes. The superior drugs, including ginseng, are absolutely nontoxic and are used for a wide variety of diseases; the middle-class drugs are effective for limited diseases and slightly toxic; the inferior or the third-class drugs are useful only for particular sicknesses and should be used with caution because of their potent activities and toxicity.[11,12]

During the Liang dynasty (about A.D. 500), a great physician, T'ao Hung-ching (A.D.452-536) was born at Mo-ling (now Nanking) and he received exceptional gifts from an early age and devoted himself to the practice of medicine.[6] He re-edited the great *Shen-nung Pen-ts'ao Ching* into *Shen-nung Pen-ts'ao Ching Chichu*. He also composed another book called *Ming-i Pieh-lu*, which contains 365 new and effective medicaments and many prescriptions that had been praised and used by many eminent physicians during the earlier Chou (1122-255 B.C.), Ch'in (255-209 B.C.), the Former Han (209 B.C.-A.D. 23), the Later Han (A.D. 25-220), and Wei (220-543) dynasties for more than one thousand years. Dr. T'ao was the first who gave the description of Chinese ginseng (from Koguryo and Paekche), their pharmacological properties, and the method of preserving them.

At the end of the Han dynasty, a system of Chinese medicine was firmly established. A well-known physician, Chang, Chung-ching, wrote his famous *Treatise on Fever*. Dr. Chang was one of the three greatest physicians of the Han dynasty. The other two outstanding doctors were Hwa, T'o, and Tsang, Kung. Dr. Chang conducted extensive clinical trials with ginseng and invented many prescriptions containing ginseng thalmologic patients were included in these two books. He was also the author of a famous medical treatise on pulse diagnosis.[13]

Up to the Sung dynasty, Liu, Han, and Ma, Chih, edited a new *materia medica* called *Kai-Pao Pen-ts'ao* with addition of 133 new medicaments. In 1057, Chang, Yu-shih, Su, Sung, *et al.* composed the well-known *Chia-yu Pen-ts'ao.* Su, Sung, himself also published *Tu-ching Pen-ts'ao* in 1061, which was the first complete dispensatory book with detailed pictorial illustrations of each medicament. In the South Sung dynasty, Ts'ao, Hsiao-ching, and others published *Cheng-ho Pen-ts'ao* in 1116, in which detailed classifications of the medicaments according to the activities of the drug were given.

Through the Tartar dynasties (916-1234) and the Yuan dynasty (1230-1341) for about four hundred years, Chinese medicine suffered a great deal as a result of wars and foreign rule.

Then in the Ming dynasty, China again recovered from foreign invasions and wars, and began to enjoy peace. The great pharmacologist and physician Dr. Li, shih-chen (1518-93), studied seriously more than eight hundred commonly encountered medicaments and traveled thousands of miles for collection of known and unknown herb medicines. He, ambitiously enough, examined the past editions of *Pen-ts'ao* written in the T'ang, Sung, and South Sung dynasties and, based on his own rich knowledge and experience gained during thirty years of uninterrupted hard work, finally composed the most monumental masterpiece in history, known as *Pen-ts'ao Kang-mu.* However, this book was not published until three years after his death. *Pen-ts'ao Kang-mu* is, in fact, an encyclopedia of naturally occurring drugs, containing fifty-two volumes in which 1,892 medicaments and 11,000 prescriptions are listed and illustrated by the aid of 1,160 figures. Among the crude drugs, 1,094 are of botanical, 444 of zoological, and the remaining of mineral origins. He classified them into sixty sections of sixteen divisions according to their source and properties. With the entry of each medicament, *Pen-ts'ao Kang-mu* gives detailed information: names, synonyms, nicknames; sources and descriptions; drug preparation and storage; prop-

erties (odor, color, taste, etc.); indications and pharmacological properties; clinical applications, contraindica-
tions, and precautions; prescriptions, formulations, and
dosage of the drug. This great writing has been praised the
world over, and starting from the seventeenth century, it has
been translated into Latin and every major Eastern and
Western language.[11]

Also during the Ming dynasty, Western civilization was introduced into China through Jesuit priests. Father Matteo Ric-
ci was the first to introduce Western medicine to the Chinese
emperor in 1601. Later in the Ch'ing dynasty (1644-1912),
most of the Western medical books and theories were introduced into China. As a result, Chinese traditional medicine then
became a disaster under the pressure of the Western powers.

From the Later Han to the Ch'ing dynasty, more than fifty
kinds (editions)of *pen-ts'ao* or dispensatories (including compendia on diet therapy) were published officially and nonof-
ficially. These represent the world's richest knowledge of herbal medicine.

It is correct to say that traditional Chinese herbal medicine is
not just a class of folk medicine. It is a well-organized medical
system developed by individual physicians and government in-
stitutions based on cumulative experience and clinical trials.

MAO'S MODERN CHINESE MEDICINE

Since the nineteenth century, the age-old Chinese civilization, of which traditional medicine was an integral part, had
started to disintegrate under the impact of Western pressure.
The Western missionary movement, specifically the Jesuits at
Peking, brought Western medicine to an isolated, feudal
China. Besides the Western missionary establishment, the
Western military, economic, and political powers forced China
(under Manchurian rule) to accept Western culture, commerce, and medicine. Particularly after the Opium War
(1839-42), all the Western powers secured a foothold in
Chinese territory. The Manchurian government (the Ch'ing
dynasty) soon collapsed, and a new government, the Republic
of China, was born in 1912.

During the Republic of China period (1912-49), however, the government's decision was to sponsor only Western medicine, while the traditional medical practice still persisted among the majority of the people, and the fate of Chinese medicine was seriously threatened and oppressed. The May Fourth movement of 1919 even denounced traditional medicine as nothing but noxious, backward, superstitious, irrational, and nonscientific, which had to be destroyed for China to survive in the modern (Western) world. Further, the government then published a decree officially prohibiting the practice of Chinese medicine. Soon civil war started, and the military Japanese invaded China. The whole country turned into a mass disaster.

The year of 1949 brought an end to the civil war with the victory of the Communist party. The new government, the People's Republic of China, without delay set up a different policy on medical practice in China that took into account the traditional art of medical practice, and, in addition, the herbal medicine and Chinese formulary was to be restudied extensively by modern scientific methods.

In 1950, Chairman Mao clearly expressed again the same medical policy that he had announced during the anti-Japanese war. In a directive to the First National Health Conference in Peking, he stressed that the Chinese should "unite all medical workers, young and old, of the traditional and Western school trained, and organize a solid united front to strive for the development of the people's health work."[14] The essence of Mao's medical thought is: (1) medical and health work should put stress on the rural areas; (2) medical services must be first for the working class; (3) practitioners of traditional Chinese medicine must be united with Western school trained doctors; and (4) health work must be integrated with mass movement. The ultimate goal of Mao's drive is to produce a unified system of modern Chinese medicine that is a marriage of traditional Chinese medicine and Western medicine.

Accordingly, the major effort on medical practice has been to send teams of urban doctors from large medical centers on periodic tours of duty in the countryside, thus providing more and better medical service for the relatively poor and neglected peasantry. Simultaneously, there has been a drive to train huge numbers of "basic level health workers," the so-called barefoot doctors for the mass population. Since the People's Republic of China was built up with the working class, to provide them with suitable medical care is essential.

It is crystal clear that Mao wanted to preserve the traditional Chinese medicine, develop it, and integrate it with modern Western medicine. On many occasions he succinctly expressed that "Chinese medicine is the summation of the experience of the Chinese people in their struggle against diseases over the past 5,000 years....Chinese medicine is a great treasure bank which must be explored and further improved with our new efforts." He further announced that "toward world health program [that the] Chinese make a great contribution is without question, one of these is the Chinese medicine."[15,16]

In addition to the new public health drive, scientific research at all levels on herb medicine as well as new antibiotics has made equal progress in the past twenty years. From 1950 to 1960, more than ten thousand scientific and clinical papers were published just on studies of herbal medicine. Few herbal medicines have antibacterial activities; the search for and manufacture of new antibiotics is similarly urgent in progress. The government is also trying to put production on a more scientific footing by growing important herbs such as *ginseng* on a plantation basis rather than depending on forest collection. In the past twenty-five years Chinese scientists have also developed a number of herbal drugs with encouraging results, for the treatment of coronary diseases, appendicitis, and gallstones, heart diseases, burns, birth control, and cancer.[17]

The Institute of Materia Medica in Peking, under the auspices of the Chinese Academy of Medical Sciences, was established in 1958 for purposes of research on new herbal drugs and new principles for common diseases. The Shanghai Institute of Materia Medica, the Institute of Organic Chemistry, and the Institue of Biochemistry in Shanghai are other leading research centers on modern Chinese medicine. The present research on herbal remedies is a national dedication to follow Chairman Mao's exhortations to explore China's herbal drugs.

Recently, Dr. E. Grey Dimond, Director of the Cardiovascular Center in Kansas City, Missouri, said on his return from his second trip to China in two years, "I was extremely impressed on the tremendous amount of information in the herb medicine. Not a cult, the Chinese had recorded and codified their herbal medicines, whereas the West had abandoned analysis of botanical medicine in favor of synthesis." Regarding the use of herb medicine for the heart-troubled patient, he said, "I have case histories of heart disease with herbal medicines being extremely effective." Finally, Dr. Dimond speculated that "I predict that herbal remedies would follow acupuncture as the next medical import from the People's Republic of China."[18]

2
GINSENG IN CHINA

For centuries, the Chinese were—and still are—the world's leading ginseng users. They value the root as a medicinal, a sort of curative charm. To the average Chinese, the value of a piece of wild ginseng root means more than gold or silver. Some authorities believe that ginseng's chief attraction for the Chinese lies in the root form, which branches out and resembles the human figure. As a matter of fact, the word *ginseng* or *Jen-shen* stems from two Chinese characters meaning *man* and *body*. The Chinese name of ginseng is often translated in Western works as *man-shaped root* or *manroot*. However, the botanist Professor S. Y. Hu of the Arnold Arboretum, Harvard University , prefers the term of *man-essence* for ginseng, since, according to Dr. Hu, ginseng was derived, on one hand, from the fanciful resemblance of the root to the human body, and, on the other hand, from the belief that this root represents the essence or elixir of the earth crystallized in a human form. Because of this, it carries the nickname of *spirit of the earth,* and sick people are relieved from their illness after taking the root. Hence, traditionally, the more the root resembles the human figure, the more potent its healing properties, and the greater its worth.

For nearly forty centuries, ginseng has been universally used in Chinese medicine as the most respected and superb health-maintaining tonic remedy. It has been prescribed repeatedly by doctors for some forty different types of illnesses in China as well as in other Asian countries. Although its mechanism remains secret, the mysterious healing power of the ginseng root is indeed a miraculous and factual truth. To the average Chinese, ginseng means medicine par excellence.[1,2]

A great deal of interest in ginseng was generated in the mid-nineteenth century in the Western world. Scientific studies on the "man-essence" were initiated in Europe, particularly in France, Germany, and the Soviet Union. Recently, Japanese and Soviet scientists, after years of laboratory and clinical investigation, have confirmed that ginseng is capable of building up vitality and physical resistance, strengthening the organism and the endocrine systems, thus overcoming illness and maintaining homeostasis. Isn't it amazing that it took nearly fifty years of endeavor to prove that the Chinese doctors' claims about ginseng's activities were basically correct?[3,4]

PANAX GINSENG: THE MOST PRECIOUS HERBAL MEDICINE

There are several varieties of ginseng in the world, the one best known being *Panax ginseng* C. A. Meyer, which is also called *Panax schinseng* Need, of the family Araliaceae. The generic name of *Panax* is derived from the Greek *pan* ($\pi\tilde{\alpha}\gamma$) meaning *all*, and *akes* (άχέουχι), meaning *cure* or *heal*. Accordingly, the word *Panax* means *cure-all, all-healing,* or *panacea*. The word *ginseng,* or *schinseng,* or more correctly *Jen-shen* or *ren-shen* in Chinese, may mean ambiguously *human body,* since the terms *gin, schin, Jen,* and *ren* all mean *man*; the terms *seng* and *shen* sound identical to *body* in Chinese.[5]

Panax ginseng is a perennial herb indigenous to the mountainous forests of Eastern Asia, particularly Eastern Manchuria (Liao-tung area), North China, Korea, and the Maritime area of Siberia. Ginseng is a very long-lived plant. Chinese *materia medica* books had claimed that only the aged ginseng root, especially the hundred- or even thousand-year-old root, gives the most potent healing power. Scientifically, this may be unfounded, but ginseng's long life is a fact. Not too long ago, the Soviet botanist Grushvitzky, found a Chinese mountain ginseng

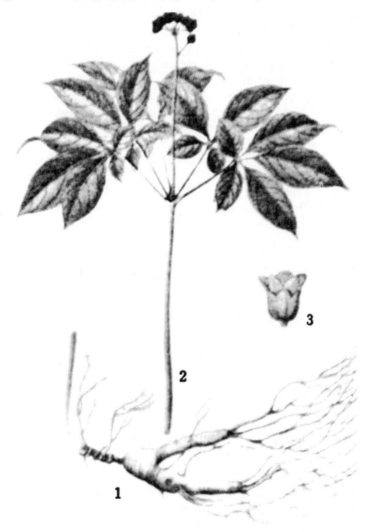

人參 （五加科）

Panax ginseng. From Handbook of Commonly Used Herbs in North China, *The People's Hygiene Publishing House, Perking 1971.*

in the Manchuria forest, and after careful examination, the root was determined to be at least four hundred years old.[6]

The Chinese believed that the best ginseng in China was the mountain-type ginseng grown only in the "Ch'ang-pai Shan"(long white mountains) area, which lies in the east of Liao-ning and south of Kirin Provinces in Manchuria. In the old days, this particular type of top-quality ginseng was extremely scarce as a result of its being difficult to collect; thus the price of it was extravagant. This particular ginseng was called *Liao-tung shen,* or *Manchurian ginseng.*

Many mountain areas in North China, however, also produce ginseng, but not *Panax ginseng.* The well-known places are Shan-si, Hopei, Shen-si, and other provinces in northern and central China. Ginseng grown in Shang-tang (now Lu-an-fu) of Shan-si, was called *Tang-shen,* and in *Tah-Kwan Pen-ts'ao,* many famous herb doctors claimed this to be the original and *genuine* Chinese ginseng with supreme healing power. Until the seventh century, both *Tang-shen* and *Panax ginseng* (Manchurian ginseng) were used widely in medicine. The original *Tang-shen* does belong to Araliaceae as can be seen from what is described in *Tah-Kwan Pen-ts'ao.*[7] However, up until the Ch'ing dynasty, the *Tang-shen* plant was classified into Campanulaceae, but no doubt the original Tang-shen has become extinct.

Three kinds of ginsng roots have been used in Chinese medicine: mountain or wild, transplanted, and cultivated ginseng. The wild ginseng grows naturally in mountains, is the most expensive, and is supposedly the most effective. Transplanted ginseng is grown from young plants moved from the mountains to farms. Cultivated ginseng is the ginseng plant grown on ginseng farms after seeding. A Chinese ginseng expert, Li, chun-chih, however, classified Chinese ginseng into six grades according to the source and age of the plant: old mountain type (over two hundred-year-old ginseng root that can only be found in Ch'ang-Pai-shen and has been praised as the most superb quality); mountain type (a few to fifty-year-old root); eradicate type (ginseng plant that was buried and revived in the mountains); transplanted type, Shih-chu ginseng (grown particularly in Kuan-hsun area); and cultivated ginseng. The experienced ginseng dealer can easily distinguish whether the ginseng is a mountain or cultivated root and can approximate the age by examining the number of rings on the surface of the root itself and the above-ground part of the plant. Mountain ginseng was very scarce even in the old days. It was said that one *catty* of Manchurian cultivated ginseng was sold at a price of two to twenty *liang* of silver or gold, while a *catty* of the aged Manchurian mountain ginseng was sold at a few thousand *liang* of silver or gold.* At such extravagant prices, genuine ginseng could hardly be afforded by the common and poor people for medicinal purposes. Naturally, only the rich, members of the emperor's families, and high officials benefited from the precious root.[5]

It is difficult to know exactly when and where the Chinese started the transplanting or growing of ginseng on farms. However, the cultivation of ginseng appeared in the poems of the T'ang and Sung dynasties. More clearly, the *Pen-ts'ao Kang-mu* recorded the method for raising ginseng on plantations. Thus it may be correct that ginseng cultivation in China started as early as the fifteenth century, but large-scale ginseng cultivation in Kirin province did not start until the eighteenth century. In Manchuria, the counties of Kuan-hsum and Juan-jen of Liaoning province, An-tu, Tun-hua, Chia-an, Fu-sung, Lin-chiang, and Wang-ch'ing of Kirin province, and Cheng-an-li of Hei-lung-kiang province are the chief areas producing wild as well as cultivated Chinese ginseng. Fu-sung is also a well-known area for cultivated ginseng. It is said that Fu-sung alone produces about sixty percent of the total ginseng in China. As a result of the constantly increasing consumption of ginseng in China, with little increase in production, the ginseng shortage remained as such for thousands of years, and China has never put great effort into cultivating on a large scale to meet her demand. Only since 1950 has the People's Republic of China put a great effort into producing the wonder root under government supervision. The most suitable conditions for growing ginseng have been under extensive study at the experimental station of She-Baa-Wang, outside of Peking.[8,9]

* One *catty* is about 1.1 pound, or 500 grams; one *liang* is about 36 grams.

A Description of Ginseng The earliest full description of the Chinese ginseng plant was given by Su, Sung, in the eleventh century. In his herbal dispensatory book *T'u-ching Pen-ts'ao*, ginseng was described as follows:

> Ginseng is grown in moist and shaded forest of Chia tree (Chia is *Tilis murensis* or *Tilia manshuria* species). The Chia tree is a broad-leaved tree, thus providing good shade. The dried ginseng seeds were planted in October as for vegetable seeds. The ginseng dies each year, and sprouts emerge in the Spring. The young plant is about 3-4 inches high with only one stem which carries five small, parted, palmate-shaped leaves. Four to five years later, it grows two stems, but still no flower stem. Until it is ten years old, it has three, later four stalks all rising from the same center, each carrying five leaflets, three large and two small. At the center of the apex of the elder plant is a flower stalk. Unlike the majority of mountain plants, ginseng has only one flower stalk which blossoms in the late spring. The ginseng blossom is small and umbrella-shaped, the size of a chestnut, and purple-white in color. It bears 7-8 seeds of soybean size after autumn. The seeds are green in color when fresh, but turn into red when ripe and drop into the ground automatically.

A Jesuit missionary in China, Fr. Jartoux, was perhaps the first Westerner who witnessed the gathering and use of ginseng in Manchuria. In a letter from Peking dated April 12, 1711 addressed to the Procurator General of the Mission of India and China, Fr. Jartoux, S.J., furnished a whole detailed description of *Panax ginseng* that he observed in Manchuria.[10]

Characteristics of Ginseng Plant Ginseng is a very slow-growing plant. The root of ginseng is collected only at a certain age of the plant and at a certain season. For example, the root is firm if it is collected in September or early October, soft if it is collected in spring or summer. The outside skin of the fresh root is yellow, but inside the skin is white. The length and diameter of the root vary with the age of the plant. It can be a few inches (a few-years old root) to a foot (after ten years). The fresh root tastes slightly bitter and somewhat sweet, and has a typical ginseng aroma.

The well-known botanist, Professor Baranov of Arnold Arboretum, Harvard University, recently published an article on morphology, cultivation, and use of ginseng.[11] The peculiar behavior of ginseng was described as:

> Not just mysterious, the ginseng root is also peculiar. It belongs to the category of contractile roots, and is an important part of a mechanism which ensures proper position for the "regeneration bud" of ginseng. The root of ginseng is normally crowned with an underground stem or vertical rhizome called the "neck". The rhizome grows upwards and increases yearly in length at the upper end. The regeneration bud is formed at the apex of the rhizome, and must necessarily find itself just at the soil-level. If the growth of the rhizome continues uncontrolled, it will finally emerge from ground and bear regeneration buds above the surface. Such a situation would be a disadvantage for the plant. Therefore, to counter-balance the lengthening of the rhizome, the ginseng root shrinks yearly at the same rate at which the rhizome grows upward, and pulls the plant downward. As a result of their mutually opposed movements, the tip of the rhizome with the regeneration bud finds itself always exactly at the soil level. This interesting morphological and biological peculiarities of ginseng plant was discovered only a few years ago.

Preparation of the Ginseng Root After the ginseng root is dug in late September or October, the root has to be treated by one of the traditional methods to make commercially acceptable and easily preserved products. There are at least six kinds of Chinese ginseng root products, prepared by six different methods.[12]

Sheng-shai shen (plain, dried ginseng) is made initially by washing and cleaning the fresh root and carefully freeing it of adhering soil without scraping the outside skin and small roots. The clean root is hung up in the air and dried completely. It is usually yellowish and slightly grey in color, with characteristic circular markings that remain untouched after this process.

Pai-kan shen (dried white ginsing) is made by cutting off the small roots and the hairy roots, scraping the outside skin from them, and drying completely in the sun. The root thus prepared is very white and smooth.

Ta-li shen (dried ginseng root) is made after carefully freeing the root from the soil, cutting off the small, the branch, and the hairy roots, then boiling briefly and drying in the sun or above a charcoal fire to complete dryness.

T'ang shen (sweetened ginseng) is made after cleaning the root, briefly boiling and puncturing the root, then putting it in syrup for about twenty-four hours. The sweetened, sugar-preserved ginseng root then is dried in the sun to complete dryness. The root thus prepared is white and sweet.

Hung shen (red ginseng) is made after carefully freeing the root of soil with a brush, cutting off the hairy and branched roots, and brushing the skin until it looks white. Then put it in a steamer to steam for about three hours. Dry it in the sun to complete dryness. The root thus prepared is semitransparent and reddish-brown in color. This is the most popular ginseng root preparation.

Shen-shu (ginseng tails) are the small ginseng roots and hairy roots that can also be made into different forms, white or red, according to the methods for the main roots.

How To Keep Ginseng Roots Ginseng roots should be kept in a dry and dark place. Since it is subject to being worm-eaten and very liable to be attacked by insects, the root must be kept in a hermetically sealed container or jar.

Adulteration Since the beginning of ginseng trade, the adulterated roots were found present and fraudulently substituted for genuine ginseng on the market. The roots of several *Campanulaceous* plants, such as *Sha-shen (Adenophora verticillata), Chi-ni (Adenophora remotifolia), Ti-ni (Adenophora tracheloides),* and *Chieh-keng (Platycodon grandiflorum),* bear close resemblance to those of ginseng and are most frequently the adulterated species. These plants and their overall pharmacological properties however, are different from ginseng. For example, the root of *Sha-shen* is more spongy and slightly cooling and demulcent. *Sha-shen* is used in Chinese medicine as an expectorant.[5] The root *Chi-ni* resembles that of *Sha-shen.* The root of *Chi-ni* is sweet and cooling. *Chi-ni* and *Chieh-keng* are botanically alike and their medicinal values are also as expectorants.[13]

THE HISTORY OF THE MANROOT

The first august sovereign and the first unifier of China, Shih Huang Ti of the Ch'in dynasty (221-209 B.C.), sought to create a durable, centralized, and unified empire that would last ten thousands of years. Legalism became the state orthodoxy. The emperor decreed the burning of all political writings and undesirable books. Toward the always dangerous enemies from the North and the West, the emperor built up the Great Wall of China, a solid, dense barrier from the sea to the west desert along the mountains that marked the northern boundaries of ancient China. The emperor also wanted longevity and immortality. Without losing any time, the emperor dispatched a group of three thousand young men and three thousand young women headed by Hsu, Fu, to the mountains in a remote eastern place that, he once heard, produced the "divine herb." This place, called Pong-lai, was later confirmed to be Japan. The divine herb that the emperor desired was said to produce rejuvenation and longevity. The supreme desire in human life is unreachable by the common man. Unfortunately this group of immortal herb collectors never returned to China, and the great emperor never had his desire of immortality fulfilled. Later people speculated the so-called miracle herb could be ginseng.[14]

During the Sui dynasty (A.D. 581-601) in the reign of Emperor Wen, the history book of *Kuang-wu Hsing-chi* records the man-shaped ginseng cry story.[1] At Shang-tang (now Lu-an of Shan-si province), at the back of a family's home each night the imploring voice of a man was heard, and nothing was found when searches were made for the source of the noise. At a distance of about a *li* (a *li* is about 3/4 mile) from the house, a remarkable plant was seen. A root was secured after digging into the ground to the depth of about five feet. The root had the shape of a man with four extremities resembling legs and arms. After this, the noise ceased, and so it was said that this plant had caused the crying out in the night with a man's voice. Thus the root was called "spirit of the ground." The mysterious nature of the man-shaped root may thus have been started.[14]

Some of the dry ginseng roots, indeed, vaguely resemble the human figure with the head (the above-ground part) on the top, and the arms and legs on the upper and lower part of the root (the side roots). It was said that the so-called man-shaped root could be made artificially by the traders or hunters. The man-shaped root usually is worth much more than the random-shaped root, which normally occurs.

In the old Chinese rural society, under the strong influence of Taoism and Buddhism, the objects encountered by the ancient Chinese people were veiled with a great deal of mystery as to their color, shape, size, smell, taste, etc., most especially so, their use as food and medicine. Wild (mountain) ginseng was believed to give better healing power than cultivated ginseng. The man-shaped ginseng root was regarded as the "divine" or "immortal" herb; after taking the root people were thought to become long-lived or "immortal."

There were quite a number of legendary stories about ginseng in ancient China. Because of the superstitious nature of the Chinese, one finds recorded in the *Pen-ts'ao Kang-mu* at least ten names, strangely enough, to describe the ginseng plant and its root.[1] *Kuei-kai*, translated as *ghost-umbrella*, means the ginseng plant is a shade (dark)-lover, and is always hiding itself from the sunshine.

Shen-ts'ao, translated as *divine herb*, means the ginseng plant has panacea power toward diseases.

Tu-ching, translated as *the spirit of the earth*, and *Ti-ching*, translated as the *spirit of the ground*, mean the mysterious nature of the ginseng root, which may be equivalent to *ghost* or *spirit of the earth*.

Shueh-shen and *Hung-shen*, translated as *blood-root* and *yellow root*, mean the ginseng root is tonic to the spleen (yellow in nature), which in turn produces blood.

Jen-wei, Jen-hsien, Hai-yu, and *Chou-mian-huan-tan* are strange names without any clear meaning.

It is difficult to know exactly when ginseng was first used in Chinese medicine. *Shen-nung Pen-ts'ao Ching* gives descriptions of ginseng and classifies it as a superior and nontoxic drug. *Ming-I Pieh-lu* has more entries about the uses of ginseng. In Chang, Chung-ching's famous medical book *The*

Treatise of Fevers, written in the Later Han dynasty (circa A.D. 195), twenty-one out of a total of 113 prescriptions contain ginseng for different ailments. Accordingly, there is no doubt that ginseng had been used as medicine in China as early as the second century,[5] or about eighteen hundred years ago.

During the Epoch of Three Kingdoms, the medicinal consumption of ginseng was much increased. The great surgeon Wa, t'o, discovered the use of ginseng in a preparation for nasal and internal bleeding.

According to another history book, *Wei-shu,* Koguryo (Kao-li), a kingdom in the northern Korean Peninsula, now North Korea and a part of Manchuria, started a diplomatic relationship with China in the third century (Wei period, 220-264). Within one hundred years, more than ninety-two diplomatic mission trips were made by the Koguryoan envoys. On each trip, the envoy brought to the Chinese emperor ginseng roots and other valuable gifts from Koguryo, and on return brought back Chinese silk, culture, and medicine. During the T'ang dynasty (618-905), the envoy from Silla (another kingdom in the southeastern part of the Korean Peninsula) made quite a number of diplomatic mission trips to China, and on five trips brought ginseng from Silla to China. The Silla ginseng roots were man-shaped, about one foot in length, wrapped in red silk, and contained in wooden boxes. However, another history book, *San-kuo Shih-chi,* recorded that once an envoy from Silla brought to the Emperor Teh of the T'ang dynasty a giant nine-foot ginseng root, but the Chinese emperor refused to receive the gift because it was not a genuine ginseng root.[14] As a result of increased communication between China and the Korean Peninsula, more ginseng roots were sold to China from Silla and Koguryo, and later the third kingdom, Packche (located in the southwestern part of the Korean Peninsula), also exported ginseng to China. In other words, since the third century, the Chinese have been keen users of Korean ginseng.

The book *Ming-I Peih-lu* gives a brief description of the Koguryoan's ginseng-hunting story. The diggers, as a rule, first prayed to their gods of the mountains for safety and good luck. After worship, as a group, they started their trip and entered the mountains with enough food, warm clothing, and arms. Conceivably, the ginseng-hunting trip was fearful and dangerous and quite often they encountered icy weather and even cruel wild animals, and no one knew if they would return alive. The people of Koguryo also have beautiful hymns to praise their mysterious divine root, which they used to call *Hsien-ts'ao,* meaning *immortal herb.* The following fabulous hymn tells how the Koguryoans searched for mountain ginseng.

> The people of Koguryo (Kao-li) praise their ginseng. The one having the three stems, five palmate leaflets, facing the shade and away from the sun is ginseng. To search for ginseng, one must discover *Tilia,* for *Tilia manshuria* always accompanies ginseng.

During the Sung dynasty, ginseng fell into seriously short supply, and the quality of ginseng and adulterated ginseng became quite a problem. One very simple method, which may be the first pharmacological test of ginseng in human history, is that according to the Su, Sung's *T'u-ching Pen-t'ao:* "In order to test for the true ginseng, two persons walk together, one with a piece of ginseng root in his mouth and the other with his mouth empty. If at the end of 3-5 *li,* the one with ginseng in his mouth does not feel himself tired, while the other is out of breath, the ginseng is genuine ginseng root".[1]

The natural ginseng plants growing in Hopei, Shan-si, and Shen-si provinces were nearly extinguished up to the Ming dynasty. Manchurian and Korean (Silla, Packche, and Koguryo) ginseng then became the only supplies available to the great demand. Korea began to export her cultivated ginseng to China during the Ch'ing dynasty at about 100,000 *catties* annually. Starting in 1875 China began to import American ginseng from the United States at about 60,000 pounds annually. As a result of the *sang* (American ginseng) boom between 1895 and 1904, an extravagant fortune was made by the ginseng diggers and traders in the United States.[15]

THE VIRTUES OF GINSENG IN CHINESE MEDICINE

Based on accumulated knowledge and experience acquired in the treament of patients during thousands of generations, doctors in the Orient, particularly in China, do believe the healing power of ginseng. Nobody realy knows how many people have been treated with the manroot in the last twenty centuries. The miraculous power of ginseng, no doubt, arises from its many therapeutically effective principles. According to classical Chinese *materia medica* books, ginseng possesses the following medicinal properties:

- a mild stimulant to the heart, nervous system, and digestive organs,
- a tonic to the impaired constitution, to add spirit, to increase digestive juices, to speed up recovery after a a long or serious illness and after a surgical operation.[5]

Ginseng is an agent that increases digestion after oral administration. It is absorbed in the small intestine, where it enters the bloodstream. It promotes blood circulation and new blood formation, thus invigorating your spirit and strengthening your body. The principal usefulness of ginseng is its *tonic* effect. It is absolutely essential to those who are suffering from diseases of consumption, neurasthenia, and its related dizziness and headache, impotence and related loss of sexual potency, impaired kidney and uterus functions, and illness due to extensive daily physical and mental activities or stresses.

In the history of Chinese medicine, the *Shen-nung Pen-ts'ao ching* was the first official medical book that stated the pharmacological virtues of ginseng.[16] The following statements are still true and universally accepted:

- tonic to the five viscera,
- quieting the spirits,
- establishing the soul,
- allaying fear,
- expelling evil effluvia,
- opening up the heart and brightening the eyes,
- benefiting the understanding,
- invigorating the body and prolonging life, if it is taken constantly.

Other famous Chinese medical treatises (see chapter 1) such as *Ming-i Pieh-lu, Hai-yao Pen-ts'ao, Yao-hsing Pen-ts'ao,* and the most famous Chinese doctor, Chang, Chung-ching's prescription books called *Wai-t'ai Mi-yao, Chia-yio Tu Ching Pen-ts'ao, Pen-ts'ao meng-ch'uan, Sih's Medical Compendium,* and Li, shin-chen's *Pen-ts'ao Kang-mu* also record the medicinal properties and different uses of ginseng.[5]

Ming-I Pieh-lu described ginseng as an effective drug for the following:

- chronic gastrointestinal disability,
- gastric and intestinal pain as a result of swelling and gas,
- dyspepsia (impaired digestion)
- difficulty in respiration,
- acute gastritis and enteritis, and vomiting,
- to increase digestive functions,
- to eliminate thirst and polyuria as a result of diabetes,
- a heart tonic, and to strengthen blood circulation,
- inflammation and swelling,
- to increase memory.

In the *Hai-yao Pen-ts'ao* ginseng was recorded to be effective in the treatment of thirst (as a result of diabetes), mental nervousness, loss of body fluid (as a result of fatigue), and to inhibit hyperchlorhydria (excess stomach acid).

Most important of all, the famous pharmacologist Li, shih-chen, after repeated testing and experimenting, listed the activities and indications of ginseng in his world-famous *Pen-ts'ao Kang-mu* as follows:

- all forms of debility of man and woman,
- various types of severe dyspepsia (impaired digestion),
- continued fever and cold perspiration,
- drowsiness and headache,
- persistant vomiting of pregnant woman,
- chronic malaria,
- exhausting discharge, polyuria, internal injuries,
- apoplexy (loss of consciousness and sensation),
- sunstroke and paralysis,
- haematemesis and menorrhagia (excessive menstrual flow),
- bleeding in feces and urine,
- hemorrhage and puerperal diseases.

The Chinese doctors, however, also warned the people *not* to abuse ginseng and *not* to take ginseng in large quantities (over one *liang*) without a prudent diagnosis by an experienced physician. Since ginseng is *not* a *placebo* but a potent remedy, its effectiveness depends upon its correct use. It is perfectly alright if you take ginseng tea or small amounts of extract every day for health-maintaining purposes, but if you are really sick, you ought not to take for granted that ginseng will be effective in the treament of certain unknown diseases, in which case it may be harmful or even hazardous.[5]

CLASSICAL GINSENG PREPARATIONS AND SECRET PRESCRIPTIONS

Ginseng can be used alone or, as a rule, used with several other ingredients in order to give a multitherapeutic or synergistic effect of healing. As mentioned in the last chapter, the "complex-remedy therapy" is the characteristic and standard practice of Chinese medicine. Ginseng extract, decoction, tincture, powder, and pills are the most commonly used ginseng preparations. According to the prescription, the drugs are weighed, mixed and a decoction or other form of preparation is made by the druggist. The dose and how often the patient has to take the preparation are also indicated in the prescription. The following are examples that explain what and how the classical Chinese ginseng preparations are usually made in typical Chinese drugstores.[17,18]

GINSENG EXTRACT *(Jen-shen Kao)* This is a watery extract made by fractionally decocting ginseng root in water and evaporating the extract to a thick liquid in a silver or earthenware pot. It was told that ginseng should never be cooked in a metal pot, except silver. The extract is normally a dark yellow or brown liquid with typical ginseng bitter-sweet taste and aroma. This extract is kept in a porcelain container.

According to the Chinese *materia medica* book *Pen-ts'ao Kang-mu,* the above ginseng extract is made in the following manner: In a silver or earthenware pot, add 10 *liang* of ground ginseng, pour into the pot 20 wine-cups of water, and soak for a little while. Then boil the infusion over a gentle flame until half of the water is evaporated. The mixture is strained (filtered) through two layers of cheese-gauze. Then put the filtrate aside. The solid portion is cooked again in the pot with 10 wine-cups of water boiling the infusion until half of the volume is reached, and filtering again. Combine the two portions of the filtrate and return them into the pot, and then boil for some time until this liquid is very thick. Store this ginseng extract in a covered porcelain container or jar.

If the extract is used for curing disease, usually it is taken once or twice a day before meals, the dose depending upon the requirement of the patient. On the other hand, for tonic purposes the above extract (containing 10 *liang* of ginseng) can be divied into 30 to 40 doses, which is the usual dose of ginseng for health-maintaining tonic effect.

Ginseng Decoction *(Jen-shen t'ang)* Most Chinese medicines are administered in the form of decoction, which is the simplest way to give medicine. It is made similarly by boiling the drug ingredients in an earthenware pot with water over a gentle flame for usually 1 to 2 hours. Unlike the extract, no further thickening is required. The decoction can be filtered, and only the liquid portion is used for medicine. The entire decotion can be administered all at once or divided into several doses depending upon the amount of drug cooked and the prescription.

Many secret prescriptions of ginseng decoction are used in China, Korea, and Japan. The following are examples of the most popular ginseng formulations for tonic effect.

Szu-chun-tze T'ang (Gentlemen's Ginseng Decoction)

Ginseng	1	*chien*	(3.6 g.)
Pai-chu	2	*chien*	(7.2 g.)
Fu-ling (Indian bread)	1	*chien*	(3.6 g.)
Licorice root	0.5	*chien*	(1.8 g.)
Fresh ginger root	2	slices	(2 g.)
Red dates	1	each	

Put the above ingredients into an earthenware pot, add water (about two cups), and bring to a boil over a gentle flame and keep boiling for some time. Strain the mixture, and use the filtrate as medicine. This particular preparation has been very widely used in China as a tonic for wasting, weakness, and tiredness.

Chih-chung T'ang (Resolvent Ginseng Decoction)

Ginseng	3 *liang*
Pai-chu	3 *liang*
Dried ginger	3 *liang*
Licorice root	3 *liang*

Put three *liang* of each of the above ingredients into an earthenware pot, and add about eight pints of water and then bring to a boil. Boil over a gentle flame for some time or until three pints remain. Strain the mixture, and the liquid portion is used. Take one pint each time, three times a day. It is a wonderful preparation for illness of the lungs, spleen, heart, and stomach.[1]

Sze-shuen T'ang (Four-Drug Decoction)

Ginseng or ginseng extract	2 *liang*
Licorice root	2 *liang*
Dried ginger	2 *liang*
Fu-tze-p'ao	2 *liang*

Add about six pints of water to the above drug ingredients in a pot and bring to a boil, boiling until the liquid is reduced to about 2.5 pints. This decoction can be divided into four doses. It has been used as a general-purpose tonic for weakness.[1]

Ch'ang-shou-t'ang (Decoction for Longevity)

Ginseng root	
Huang-chi (Yellow vetch)	
Pai-chu	1 *chien*
Tu-chung	
Niu-hsi (Ox knee)	
White peony	
Licorice root	0.6 *chien*

Wu-wei-tze	12 pieces
Shu-ti-huang	2 *chien*
Red dates	1 each

In a similar manner the above drug ingredients are made into a decoctin. Taken before meals, it serves as a potent tonic for good health and longevity.[17]

A decoction used for restorative purposes is made with ginseng extract, orange peel tincture, and ginger juice, each of suitable amount, taken before meals.

Another decoction used for restorative purposes is made with ginseng extract, orange peel tincture, and honey, each of a suitable amount. Mix them together, and drink it before going to bed.

GINSENG TINCTURE *(Jen-shen chiu)* Traditionally, tinctures are made by macerating the ground drug in a mixture of rice and leaven during the process of fermentation for producing spirit. However, the modern method of making tincture can be achieved by extracting the drug with wine or spirit to give an alcoholic tincture. The ginseng tincture preparation has been made in Chinese dispensatories, but it is not as popular as ginseng decoctions. However, the ginseng tincture mixed with tincture of *Kou-chi (Lycium Chinense)* and/or tincture of *Lu-jung (Moaochasme savatieri)* has been used for tonic purposes, especially, for sexual debility and impotence in males.[5]

GINSENG POWDER *(Jen-shen San)* The powdered ginseng root or the dried ginseng extract can be used as tea or soup, to drink alone or with another substance such as sugar or honey. This is a tonic of choice for those who have peptic ulcers and are unable to take ordinary drinks of coffee or tea.

GINSENG PILLS *(Jen-shen Wan)* In Chinese medicine, pills have been widely used and are a favorite solid preparation for exhibiting drugs without exposing disagreeable tastes to the patient. Pills are generally divided into *Wan, Tan,* and *San,* made in all sizes from that of a millet seed to that of a pigeon's egg. Pills are usually coated with some typical coating materials to mask the bitter taste. Rice flour and honey are the most widely used fillers in making pills. Among hundreds of pill preparations in Chinese medicine, the following are some of the most popular ginseng pill formulations.

Tsao-shen Wan (Date Ginseng Pills)

These are made of large Chinese red dates and ginseng extract. They are said to be useful in strengthening the respirative organ.

Chen-Jen Pao-Ming Tan (Sour-date Ginseng Pills)

These are made of *Suan-tsao (zizyphus jujuba),* ginseng, *Fu-ling,* and *T'ien-men-tung,* three *chien* of each, soaked with wine or spirit for some time (three days). Then the alcoholic extract is evaporated to dryness and made into pills. Take one-fourth of the total pills before going to bed. They are used for increased sexual potency.[18]

Jen-shen Kwie-pi Wan (Ginseng Cinnamon Pills)

Mix powdered ginseng, *Jou-kuei* (fleshy cinnamon), *Mai-men-tung, Wu-wei-tzu,* and other excipients to make pills. It is said that this preparation has been used traditionally in the Orient as an aphrodisiac.[5]

OTHER USEFUL HERB MEDICINES The ingredients besides ginseng in the above formulations serve as minor tonic, curative, supplementary, or flavoring agents. They may also give synergistic action or nullify the possible interactions between the ingredients. These ingredients are used over and over again in almost every tonic preparation in Chinese medicine. The following are brief descriptions of these most commonly used ingredients in ginseng prescriptions.[1,5]

Fu-ling (Pachyma cocos)

This is an Asian herb. It is a fungus growth upon the roots of fir trees. It has been used as food and medicine. It is considered to be a septic, diuretic, and calmative, especially in the nervous disorders of children. It is also a tonic to cure chest pain and invigorate the body.

Cassia bark (Cinnamon cassia)

This is native to Kwang-si province and other parts of southern China. It is more often used as a condiment than a medicine, being employed as a flavoring agent for Chinese cooking of meats. Medicinally it is a stomachic, stimulant, carminative, astringent, sedative, and tonic.

Pai-shu (Atractylis)

This is largely grown in southern China. The dried roots are used medicinally. It is a stomachic, stimulant, arthritic, tonic, and diuretic remedy used in fever, catarrh, chronic dysentary, general dropsy, rheumatism, profuse sweating, and apoplexy. It has been widely used in tonic formualtions.

Ginger (Zingiber officinale)

Both fresh and dried ginger root have been used in Chinese medicine. It is a pungent, aromatic, stimulant, and carminative to expel gas from the stomach and bowel.

Licorice root (Glycyrrhiza globra)

This is the most commonly used herb sweetener in Chinese medicine in preparations for cough remedies, and serves as a soothing emollient in preparations designed to treat the chest and lung disorders.

Mai-men-tung (Ophiopogon spicatus)

The root is the part used in medicine. It is nontoxic and edible. It has some of the properties of squill. It is supposed to benefit the dual principles and is, therefore, tonic and aphrodisiac promoting fertility.

Red dates *(Zizyphus vulgaris)*

These are commonly cultivated jujube. They are grown in northern and southern China. They are much used in food, especially in the preparations of confections. They are considered nourishing, beneficial to the viscera, tonic, quieting and laxative.

T'ien-men-tung *(Asparagus lucidus)*

This is produced in North China. It has the taste of squill. It is considered to be an expectorant, tonic, stomachic, and nervous stimulant. Prolonged use is recommended in impotence.

Wu-wei-tzu *(Schizandra chinensis)*

This drug is said to have five distinct tastes. The skin and pulp of the fruit are sweet and sour, the kernels are pungent and bitter, and the whole fruit has a salty taste. This gives rise to the name *five flavors*. Medicinally it is a tonic, aphrodisiac, with pectoral and lenitive properties.

OTHER MIRACULOUS ROOTS AS GINSENG SUBSTITUTES

There are at least eight medicinal plants that are cousins of *P. ginseng*. Because the roots of these plants bear close resemblance in action to ginseng, they also carry the general name of *shen*, and they have been widely used in the Orient for ginseng substitute. Each of them occupies a particular place in Chinese medicine.[1,5] They are: *Sha-shen, Hsuan-shen, Tan-shen, Kú-shen, Tzu-shen, Tai-tzu-shen, Tang-shen,* and *Jen-shen-san-ch'i.* Though these roots are less well known than ginseng, they are equally useful medicinally, and their prices are much lower.

It was recorded as early as in *Ming-I-Pieh-Lu,* that five miraculous remedies, more correctly called *Wu-shen,* were known in Chinese medicine. The *Wu-shen* are: *Jen-shen*, (ginseng), *Sha-shen*, *Hsuan-shen*, *Tan-shen*, and *Kú-shen*. None of these five remedies belongs to the same family botanically. However, the five slightly different plants were grouped together by Li, Shih-chen. Thus, the *Wu-shen* are: *Jen-shen* (ginseng), *Sha-shen*, *Hsuan-shen*, *Tan-shen*, and *Tzu-shen*.

It is very interesting to note that the dried roots of each of these species carries a particular color, and thus it was assumed that each of the plants may act specifically upon each of the principal five viscera. Certainly this complies with ancient Chinese medical thinking. *Jen-shen* has been claimed to act chiefly upon the spleen, the center of life. Being yellow in color, *Jen-shen* has been called *Huang*(yellow)-*shen*; *Sha-shen*, grown in sand-soil, is much whiter than *Jen-shen* (ginseng), and is also called *Pai*(white)-*shen*. It acts principally upon the lungs; *Hsuan-shen* is also called *Hei*(black)-*shen*. Because its root, stem, and seeds are dark or nearly black, it is supposed to act on the kidney; *Tan-shen*, being red in color, is also called *Ch'ih*(red)-*shen*. It acts on the heart and the blood. *Tan-shen* has been highly recommended in all blood difficulties such as hemorrhages, menstrual disorders, and miscarriages. *Tzu-shen*, also called *Mou-meng*, is purple in color and acts chiefly upon the liver. It has been prescribed for kidney and blood disorders.[19] The truth of these medicinal claims needs scientific confirmation, and little data is available at present.

Sha-Shen *Sha-shen* has also been called *Yang-ru* (goat milk) in addition to *Pai*(white)-*shen*. Its root gives milky white juices, and it is much whiter than the *Jen-shen* root. Botanically, *Sha-shen* is *Adenophora verticillata* of the family Campanulaceae. The best *Sha-shen* was from the Hwa-shan area in China. Natural and cultivated *Sha-shen* are now grown in the southeast and the north of Sze-chwan provinces of China. The root of *Sha-shen* tastes slightly bitter and cool. It has been used for pulmonary disorders, especially those attended by fever and cough, and it is used as a general tonic and restorative agent. *Jen-shen* and *Sha-shen* have been prescribed selectively for different symptoms. For lung disorders with burning, *Sha-shen* was used; for lung disorders with cooling, *Jen-shen* was used. It was said that *Sha-shen* is a tonic for the yin, while *Jen-shen*, a tonic for the yang of the five viscera.[19]

Hsuan-Shen *Hsuan-shen* has also been called *Yeh-chih-ma* in addition to *Hei*(black)-*shen*. Botanically it is called *Scrophularia Oldhami,* Oliv. It blossoms in March, grows about four to five feet high, and has a slender stem that resembles that of ginseng. It has opposite leaves, long and serrated, resembling those of wild sesame. It bears black seeds, and also greenish-blue or white flowers in August. The root and stem of *Hsuan-shen* has a fishy odor.

The root tastes slightly bitter and cooling. It has been used as a tonic, restorative, and diuretic. It also has been used in stomach and intestinal fevers, malaria, extreme thirst, abcess, scrophulous glands, and galactorrhoea.[1,20]

Tan-Shen *Tan-shen* has also been called *Chu-ma* or *Beng-ma ts'ao* in addition to *Ch'ih*(red)-*shen*. Botanically, it is *Salvia miltiorrhiza* Bunge of the family Labiatae. It is now grown in the Ho-pei, Shan-tung, An-hwei, Szu-chẃan, and Kiang-su provinces of China.[1,21]

It sprouts in February and grows to about one foot high with opposite leaves that resemble those of peppermint leaves. It has purple blossoms starting in April and bears red fruit.

It has been prescribed for many blood disorders, particularly menstrual ailments, miscarriages, and hemorrhages. It stimulates blood circulation and the formation of blood cells. It has also been used for beriberi, joint pains and arthritic ailments, nervous insomnia, enlargement of the spleen, and hypertension.[22]

In animal health, *Tan-shen* has been used for horses, stimulating racing horses for prolonged activities and better performance.[1]

K'u-Shen *K'u-shen* has also been called *K'u-shih* or *K'u-kuo* (bitter bone), *k'u* meaning *bitter* in Chinese. Botanically, it is *Sophora angustifolia* of the family Leguminosae. It is a very common plant in central China and Manchuria. It bears yellowish-white flowers, a siliquaceous pod, and it has a long yellowish and exceedingly bitter root. The best species is from the Ho-nan province of China.[23]

K'u-shen has been given in stomach disorders, indigestion, jaundice, fevers, dysentery, leprosy, scrofula, and leucorrhea.[23]

Tzu-Shen Another name of *Tzu-shen* is *Mou-meng*. Botanically it is *Polygonum bistorta* of the family Polyganaceae. It has purple-white blossoms in May, and bears black seeds. It has a purple-black root with a bitter and cool taste.[1]

It has been used as a tonic, an antifebrile, a diuretic, and a laxative. It has also been prescribed for internal and external hemorrhages, anemorrhaea, agus, and dysentery.[24]

Tai-Tzu-Shen Botanically it is called *Pseudostellaria rhaphanorrhiza* Pax. of the Caryophyllaceae family. It has also been called *Tzu*(baby)-*shen*. It is produced mainly in the Kiang-su province of China. It has been used as a ginseng substitute for tonic action.[25]

Tang-Shen There are many varieties of *Tang-shen* in China, but the most important one is botanically *Condonopsis tangshen* Oliv. of the family Campanulaceae. It is produced mainly in the Shan-si, Shen-si, Ho-pei, and Kan-su provinces of China. It was used as a ginseng substitute.[25]

3

KOREAN GINSENG

HIGHLIGHTS OF KOREAN GINSENG

Korean ginseng is botanically identical to the ginseng plant growing in Manchuria and in the maritime province of Siberia. In the old days, Korean ginseng plants grew abundantly in the forestal mountains over the peninsula. Wild mountain ginseng is called *san-sam*. Korean ginseng has been a very valuable remedy in medicine since the sixth century. In modern times, Korea has become the major ginseng-producing country in the world. This may be ascribed to the fact that Korea has the longest history in producing ginseng. Moreover, the climate and geographical conditions may provide an optimum condition for ginseng cultivation. Korea deserves the title of the "ginseng country."

According to legend, Korean history began some four thousand years ago. The majority of the Korean people were immigrants from North China and Manchuria. About A.D. 100 the kingdom of Koguryo, the first truly Korean state, emerged in the middle Yalu region. During the fourth century, the tribes of the southern half of the peninsula had coalesced into three federations, known as the Three Han. Paekche in the southwestern or Ma Han area, and Silla in the southeastern, or Pyon Han region, and the Chin Han region, which lay across the center of the peninsula, fell to the hands of Koguryo in the early fifth century. In the ensuing struggle among the Three Kingdoms of Koguryo, Paekche, and Silla, it was Silla that won

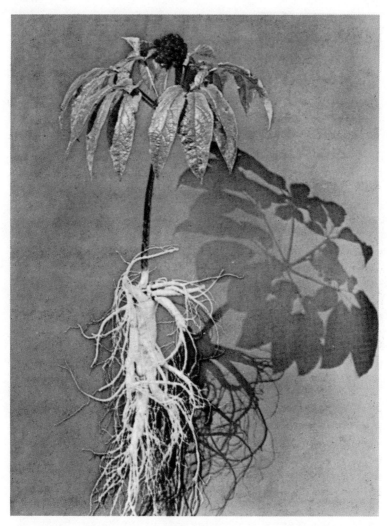

Ginseng.

control of the peninsula under the help of the Chinese army during T'ang dynasty. Then came the Silla Unification Period. During the Yi dynasty (1392-1910), King T'aejo adopted the name of Chosen for Korea, and moved the capitol from Kaesong to Seoul. The dynasty he established lasted five hundred years until the annexation of Korea by Japan.[1]

As a result of the historic close association between Korea and China, Chinese medicine was prevelent in Korea, and Korean ginseng was known to the Chinese as early as in the third century (during the Wei dynasty). Even in the very beginning, the Koguryo kingdom envoys made ninety two diplomatic trips to China, and each time Koguryo ginseng was brought to the Chinese emperor as the most valuable gift. In the sixth (Sui dynasty) and seventh to ninth centuries (T'ang dynasty), ginseng roots from Paekche and Silla were similarly offered to the Chinese emperors on numerous occasions. Ginseng root was used by emperors and high officials in ancient China as the most valuable medicine.

According to Chinese medical literature, the three different types of ginseng (root) from the Three Kingdoms are not all equal in appearance, color, taste, and activity. The great Chinese physician Tao, Hung-ching recorded the descriptions of the ginsengs in his book as follows: "The ginseng (root) from Paekche is slender, round in shape, firm and with lighter taste than that of *tang-shen* (the genuine ancient Chinese ginseng); ginseng from Koguryo is large, soft, and inferior to *tang-shen* and that from Paekche. The ginseng from Silla is yellowish with light taste, and more closely resembles the human figure."[2]

Cultivation of Korean Ginseng Growing ginseng plants was first started in the Ching-shan and Chuan-lo provinces in South Korea in the sixteenth century. Later ginseng was cultivated on large scales in Kei-jo (Kae-song) and Kum-san. New ginseng cultivation centers are Kang-gye, Kum-kand, Kyang-ji, Chung-chu, and Che-ju. In the beginning of the twentieth century, the production of Korean ginseng reached 700,000 pounds per year, valued at more than two million yen. Most of this was exported to China, Japan, and other southeastern

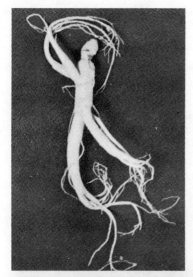

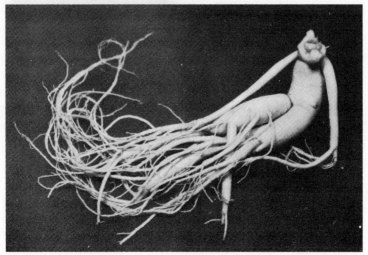

Ginseng.

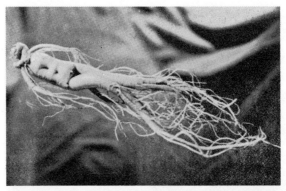

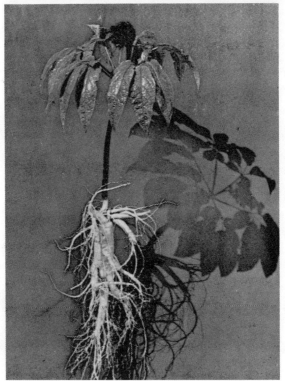

Ginseng.

Asian countries. Even at that time, the top-grade Korean red ginseng root was sold at about $30-35 per *catty*, which was about seven times higher than the price of imported American ginseng, or about twice that for Korean white ginseng.[3]

Unfortunately, a disastrous effect of the ginseng disease that broke out in 1902 in Korea crippled the business for about eleven years and threatened to extinguish the entire trade, and there were no exports until 1910.[4]

The climate and soil of the Korean Peninsula are peculiarly suited for ginseng cultivation. More and more farmers attempted to grow ginseng plants for higher profit. At present there are thirty-three ginseng-growing districts in South Korea including Kang-wha, Kim-po, Kum-san, and Pu-yo whose annual production of crude ginseng amounts to 5,700,000 kg. The figures is expected to be increased to fifteen million kg. in 1981 according to the Korean Office of Monopoly. The total cultivation area of red ginseng products is about sixteen million square meters. With such industrialized cultivation, a supply shortage in ginseng is not expected in the next ten years in Korea's ability to support the world market.[5]

Ginseng Law Korea has a long history in governing and controlling ginseng production, particularly the red ginseng root. The control of the production and sale of red ginseng was initiated in the seventeenth century (the Yi dynasty, A.D. 1606). Probably the first government regulation of ginsent was promulgated in 1686 and the second in 1707. From 1897 to 1910, red ginseng production and trade were controlled directly by the emperor's office. In 1868 taxation on ginseng cultivation in the Gae Seung area was begun.

A so-called modern monopoly law and its bylaws for red ginseng were established in 1907. There were revisions in these laws in 1920, and they were effective until 1945. The major regulations of the ginseng monopoly law included registration of seeds, and intensifying the penalty for illegal production of red ginseng. During the Japanese annex period (1910-45), the Office of Monopoly, located in Kaesong, was controlled by the Japanese.

In August 15, 1947, Korea was divided into South and North Korea. The famous ginseng city Kaesong was divided into two parts. As a result of social instability, ginseng production was suspended for quite a number of years. Fortunately, Korean ginseng production has been revitalized since 1960. In order to promote the quality of ginseng and its products uniformly, the monopoly law of red ginseng of December 1959 was radically revised in December 1972. A new regulation on white ginseng and its products was simultaneously promulgated. The production and sale of white ginseng products then became privately owned operations that were also subject to control by the 1972 ginseng law.[3]

REMEDIAL USE OF GINSENG IN KOREA

Although ginseng has been recognized by the Koreans as a useful remedy dating back to the Three Kingdom period, it became a recognized medicine only in the Yi dynasty. Ginseng was used in Korea, as in China, for its alternative, tonic, stimulant, carminative and demulcent properties. It has reputed virtues for all forms of debility and dyspepsia, spermatorrhea, persistent vomiting of pregnancy, old cough, and polyuria, which are treated with ginseng preparations for relief and cure.[4]

In the early tenth century, ginseng was also used in making food and cosmetic products. Ginseng drinks, tea, candy, and cosmetics preparations, such as toothpaste, bath oil, and creams, were the most commonly processed ginseng preparations.

Ginseng's tonic effect has also been tested in the veterinary field. It was said that in the sport of horse racing, ginseng was given in the horses' feed for about several weeks before racing. The horses under ginseng treatment showed better performance than those without.[6]

MODERN KOREAN GINSENG PRODUCTS

Ginseng root as it is dug up is called watery ginseng (*su-sam*) from which white ginseng root (*pae-sam*), yellow ginseng root (*hwang-sam*), and red ginseng root (*hong-sam*) are processed. White ginseng root is made by initially peeling the watery root with a bamboo knife after it has been cleaned, and drying it in the sun, or when the weather is unfavorable, drying over a

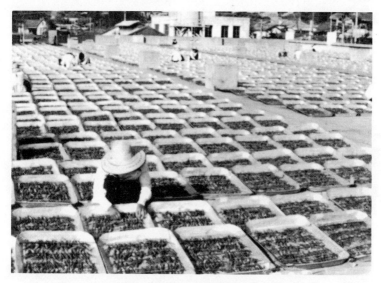

Sun-dried raw ginseng.

charcoal fire or in an oven. Yellow ginseng is made by steaming the peeled watery root and then drying it. This type of product is less desirable. The making of red ginseng root includes steaming the watery root for about three to four hours, dehydrating it in a dry room, and parching it in the sun. Red ginseng is monopolized by the Korean government and cultivators are prohibited from making and selling it. White

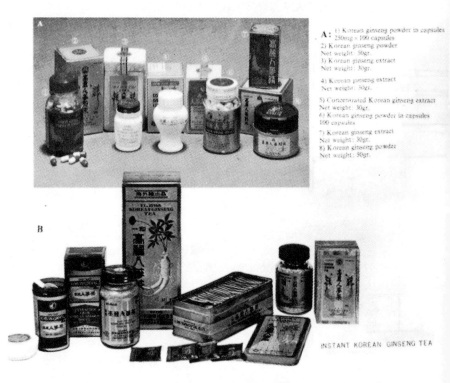

A: 1) Korean ginseng powder in capsules
250mg × 100 capsules
2) Korean ginseng powder
Net weight: 50gr.
3) Korean ginseng extract
Net weight: 50gr.

4) Korean ginseng extract
Net weight: 30gr.

5) Concentrated Korean ginseng extract
Net weight: 30gr.
6) Korean ginseng powder in capsules
100 capsules

7) Korean ginseng extract
Net weight: 30gr.
8) Korean ginseng powder
Net weight: 50gr.

INSTANT KOREAN GINSENG TEA

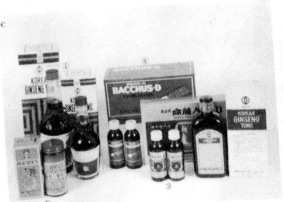

C: 1) Korean Ginseng Tonic
375ml, 500ml, 750ml/bt.
Nutritional liquid for general asthenia contains Korean ginseng extract and other active principles of various Chinese herbs
2) Korean Ginseng Tea
100gm/bt.
Finely granulated instant tea contained 8% of ginseng extract
3) Korean Ginseng Drink
100ml/bt.
Refreshing drink which contains 0.3% of ginseng extract
4) Bacchus D-ginseng fortified Drink
100ml/bt.
Nutritional and refreshing drink which contains ginseng extract, essential amino acid and vitamins

Korean ginseng products.

ginseng looks slightly yellowish-white, while red ginseng is somewhat translucent and reddish-brown in color. Both red and white ginseng are packaged in sealed cartons marked with name, grade, total weight, number of roots, and source of production printed on the box.[7]

Modern ginseng products are being developed to meet the government standards for exportation. The newer products are honey ginseng, ginseng extract, ginseng powder, ginseng pills, ginseng capsules, ginseng tablets, ginseng tea, ginseng syrup, ginseng cakes and candies, ginseng tincture, ginseng elixir, ginseng fluid extract, and ginseng alcoholic beverage.[8] The most popular ginseng tonic preparations, such as ginseng in wine (*In-sam-Ju*), ginseng chicken essence, ginseng concentrate, and ginseng-vitamin-mineral combination preparations, are presently the most desirable marketed products.

White Ginseng Root

This is one of the most popular ginseng products of South Korea to date. It is packaged into 600g., 300g., 150g., and 75g. boxes. The largest roots weigh about 47 g. per piece, the medium-sized roots weigh about 10 g. per piece, and the smallest roots weigh only 3 g. per piece. As a result of the sizes, the price of the white ginseng varies significantly.

Honey Ginseng

This is white ginseng root preserved in syrup. It gives a palatable taste.

Ginseng Tea

The instantly soluble granules are packaged in foil bags or in bottles. The granules contain about eight percent of dry ginseng extract and soluble inert materials such as lactose and soluble starch. It gives a stimulant effect with typical ginseng flavor and fragrance.

Ginseng Extract

This is the most potent ginseng product for tonic effect. It contains about forty percent of water, and sixty percent solid materials including extracted principles from the root.

Ginseng Capsules

These contain dried ginseng extract and inert fillers.

Cosmetics and Animal Health Products

In the cosmetic area, creams and beauty lotions have been marketed for rejuvenation and a young-looking effect. In the field of animal health, ginseng, can also be used in many cases for an antifatigue effect, and homeostasis, and may produce longevity as well.

4
GINSENG IN JAPAN, SIBERIA, AND THE HIMALAYAS

GINSENG IN JAPAN AND *CHIKUSETSU NIN-JIN*

The beginning of the Yamato era in the third century marked the unification of ancient Japan. At the time, Japan was a young, struggling country, while her neighbor, China, had been enjoying a highly developed culture and social life. The Yamato government sent the first envoy to China in 607, and thus established a diplomatic relationship with the emperor of the Sue dynasty. Later in the T'ang dynasty, the Japanese government dispatched students, monks, and professionals as well as envoys to China to observe and learn Chinese culture and technology. After the Taike reform in 645, Japan adopted the Chinese written language, art, crafts, social and government systems, and medicine. In 710, the first permanent capitol, Heijo (later called Nara), was built after T'ang's capitol of Ch'ang-an. In the Japanese society, it became stylish to copy the gorgeous silk robes worn by the Chinese nobility, and to imitate their custom and social manners.[1] Chinese medicine was adopted and practiced in Japan, known as Kan-po-I in Japanese. Chinese medicine occupies a special place in Japan even today.

Nin-jin, means ginseng, while *Panax ginseng* is called *Otane-ninjin* in Japanese. Though ginseng has been imported to Japan from Korea (the Kingdom of Paekche) and China in the seventh century, ginseng started to be used as a medicine in the eighth century. At that time, ginseng was the most valuable drug and it was controlled by a special office of the emperor. The price of ginseng was extremely high, and it was available only to the palace, nobles, and the rich. Ginseng became more popular after the ninth century due to more Korean ginseng being available. Chinese medicine in Japan became the flourishing medical practice after the ninth century, and lasted for about one thousand years until the Meiji restoration in 1868.

In the early Japanese medical practice, ginseng was used for tonic, stomachic, many forms of debility, cardiac stimulant, thirst, diabetes, vomiting, coolness of limbs, etc. It was used alone or with other drugs as in the popular prescriptions in Chinese medicine. Ginseng was used in many special preparations, such as cosmetics, drinks, tea, candy, and in preparations, for aphrodisiac properties with deer's antlers, cinnamon, seal's kidney, and musk, as described in the Japanese books *Nin-Jin-Shih (History of Ginseng)*.[2]

There is no evidence that Japan had wild mountain ginseng in ancient times. Japan imported ginseng seeds from Korea in 1607, and later a large amount of seeds, seedlings, and even live roots were imported from Korea and China and planted in quite a number of counties in Japan where the weather, soil, and terrain were suitable. Hokkaido, Yamagata, Nagano, Shimane, and Fukushima were the early ginseng cultivation centers. Ginseng was called "Imperial ginseng," and after a few failures, ginseng farming finally succeeded. In 1907, ginseng cultivation became a good business, and thousands of farmers grew ginseng, which was distributed in forty-three counties. However, this boom did not last too long, a ginseng epidemic occurred, and most of the farms then died away.[3]

In modern times, ginseng in Japan is cultivated in Fukushima, Nagano, and Shimane counties. In the beginning, the annual production of ginseng in Japan was about 70,000 kg. to 200,000 kg. The latest Fuji marketing report shows that growing ginseng is still a fairly profitable business. Ginseng farmers are not growing ginseng exclusively, but are regular rice growers. From 1969 to 1975, the ginseng farming areas were increased from 383 hectares in 1969, to 413 hectares in

1972, to 425 hectares in 1975, although the number of farms were actually decreased from 4,590 in 1969, to 4,040 in 1972. Most of the ginseng farms are small, individual gardens, and about eighty percent of the total 4,000 — 5,000 farms are located in Nagano county. Collective cultivation of ginseng was only recently conducted in Shimane county.[4]

The actual ginseng cultivation areas in the three counties in 1973 were: 82 hectares (19 percent) in Fukushima, 250 hectares (58.5 percent) in Nagano, and 96 hectares (22.5 percent) in Shimane county. (One hectare is 2.47 acre). The total ginseng farming area in Japan is about 1,057 acres.

The total annual production is about 319,000 kg. or 703,267 lbs. divided into 54,000 kg from Fukushima, 185,000 kg. from Nagano, and 80,000 kg. from Shimane county. Accordingly, the production of ginseng in Nagano alone is about fifty-eight percent of the total ginseng produced in Japan.

The fresh ginseng roots are processed to make commercially useful products. The majority of the roots are made into red ginseng according to the classical Chinese methods, and exported to China and Hong Kong. The rest of them are made into white ginseng and other processed products for domestic consumption and exporting.

In the early twentieth century, Japan had no problem in getting Chinese and Korean ginseng, for she annexed Korea to her protectorate in 1907, and later occupied Manchuria in 1923 until the end of World War II in 1945. During the Japanese military occupation of the ginseng country and ginseng-rich Manchuria, the entire ginseng business was monopolized by the Japanese government. Also during the occupation years, Japanese scientists made serious studies of ginseng.

Chikusetsu nin-jin, or Japanese ginseng, has been native to the mountain areas of Japan since ancient times. The word *chikusetsu* means that the ginseng root resembles that of bamboo knots. Botanically, it is *Panax japonicum* C. A. Meyer, of the Araliaceae family. It has also been called To-jin, meaning *native ginseng,* and *tochiba ninjin,* in Japanese.

The Japanese ginseng plant above ground part is very similar to *Panax ginseng,* but the root is not. Japanese ginseng root tastes more bitter than ginseng, and it is much cheaper. For thousands of years, Japanese ginseng has been used as a ginseng substitute for an expectorant, stomachic, and antipyretic agent in the Orient.

GINSENG IN SIBERIA

Panax ginseng also is found naturally in the maritime areas of Siberia. In ancient times, ginseng grew over vast territories. At present, it grows in considerable amounts only in the territories of the Soviet Union, where state laws prevent it from extermination. A special state farm called *Zhenshen* has been founded to grow this most valuable medicinal plant. Scientific establishments and individual ginseng growers in the Caucasus, and the Ukraine, in the Baltic republic, and in Siberia have also amassed a vast experience in growing ginseng.[5]

Eleuthero, botanically known as *Eleutherococcus senticosus* Maxim of the Araliaceae family, is called *Siberian ginseng* under the popular name. Because its branches are spiked with thorns, it has nicknames of *touch-me-not* and *devil's bush*. Siberian ginseng is not known in Oriental medicine, although it is abundant in eastern Siberia, in Korea, and even in the provinces of Shan-si and Ho-pei of northern China. But the naturally growing area of *Eleuthero* in Siberia exceeds ten million hectares.[6]

It is a shrub about two meters in height with numerous thin thorns. The leaves are long stalked, palmately parted, and similar to those of ginseng. The flowers are small (female is yellow, male is violet in color) gathered in globular umbrellae. It blooms in July, and bears oval fruit; the fruit turns black when ripened in September.

Scientific studies on *Eleuthero* in the Soviet Union found that Siberian ginseng is of negligible toxicity and has anabolic,gonadotropic, stimulating, protective, and adaptogenic action. One of the possible mechanisms of numerous useful effects of the Siberian ginseng preparations is the antistress action.[7] In this regard, Siberian ginseng is very similar to *Panax ginseng*.

HIMALAYAN GINSENG and *San-Ch'I* Ginseng *(Jen-Shen-San-Ch'I)*

The Himalaya Mountains, often called the Roof of the World, lie in the heart of Asia. The majestic Himalayas are about 1,500 miles long and 150 miles wide. The glorious Mount Everest at 29,028 feet is the world's highest mountain, and more than forty other awesome peaks similarly soar skyward to over 25,000 feet. Little is known about most of the mountainous land, but natives speak of evil spirits and gods living on the higher peaks and ridges. There are also legends of the Abominable Snowman, which add to the mystery of the area.

Above 12,000 feet, the timberline vanishes. Roaring winds, heavy snows, and freezing temperatures make life hard for people and animals who live at this elevation. However, in the mountainous forest, Himalayan ginseng was found in the eastern Himalayas.[8] It is said that the Himalayan ginseng is very similar to *San-ch'i* ginseng and Japanese ginseng *(P. japonicum* C. A. Meyer), and botanically it belongs to *Panax pseudoginseng* sub sp. himalaicus var. angustifolius of Araliaceae. This newly discovered ginseng plant has been investigated by Professors H. Harra of Tokyo University, N. Kondo of Showa University, and O. Tanaka of Hiroshima Unversity.[9]

Jen-shen-san-ch'i (San-ch'i ginseng) has also been called *Shan-ch'i (meaning a mountain varnish),* or *Chin-pu-huan* (meaning *a precious drug)* in Chinese. Botanically it is called *Panax pseudoginseng* Wallich, of Araliaceae. This perennial plant is named for the irregular growth of its leaves. It was said that there were three leaflets on the right and four leaflets on the left of the stem, and they grew directly out of the apex of the stem. But this is not the description of Jen-sen-san-ch'i today.[10]

This plant grows naturally and is cultivated in the southwestern part of China. The primary area of natural production is in the forest mountains of the southeastern Yun-nan province and its adjacent areas of Kwang-si province, on the slopes of one thousand to two-thousand meters, particularly in

Wen-shan, Kwang-nan, Hsi-chow, and Yen-shan in Yun-nan province and Tien-gang and Chig-hsi in Kwang-si province. About ninety percent of the commerical product of *San-ch'i* ginseng today is from Yun-nan province. For this reason, the crude drug has been called *Yun-nan San-ch'i*. However, the *San-chi* has also been cultivated on slopes at altitudes of one thousand meters and above of Kwang-si and Yun-nan provinces. Loose acid soil, rich in humus is preferred. The natural plant of *San-ch'i* ginseng can also be found in Sze-chwan, King-si provinces of China, North Vietnam, the Himalayas, and northern India.

The growth habit of *Jen-shen-San-ch'i* is similar to ginseng's. The crude drug is the properly dried root of four to six-year-old plant. The root of *San-ch'i* ginseng is fleshy, firm, round or conical in shape, with a smooth skin, brownish gray in color, and the root is about two to four centimeters long and one to two centimeters in diameter. It tastes bitter first then slightly sweetish.[10]

Pharmacologically *Jen-shen-san-ch'i* is a very effective agent in arresting hemorrhage and bleeding in wounds, including snake and tiger bites. Internally, it has been prescribed in haematenesis, menorrhagia, etc. The leaves also have similar properties and are often combined with the root for medicinal preparations. It is said that the famous secret formula of *Yun-nan-Pai-yao* (a famous pharmaceutical antibleeding preparation made in Yun-nan province) contains the active principles of this particular plant as the effective constituent. Chemical studies of *Jen-shen-san-chi* have been carried out in China as well as in Japan in the past. It was found that this plant contains saponin glycosides of Arasaponin A ($C_{17}H_{30}O_5$) and Arasaponin B ($C_{29}H_{32}O_3$) as the principal active agents. The total alcoholic extract of crude saponins has been reported to be twelve percent. At the present, we do not know whether *San-ch'i* ginseng also contains the other principles found in Himalayan ginseng.[10,11]

5
AMERICAN GINSENG

The ginseng plant found in North America is commonly called American ginseng and is only slightly different from the one native to China. American ginseng is also called *sang, red berry,* and *five fingers.* Botanically, it is known as *Panax quinquefolium* Linn. of the Araliaceae family named by Linnaeus in 1753. It is a fleshy, rooted, perennial herbaceous plant.

In the old days, it grew naturally on the slopes of ravines and in other shady but well-drained areas in hardwood forests from Quebec to Manitoba, and from Maine and Minnesota southward to the mountains of Georgia, Arkansas, and Louisiana. The properly dried roots were used as remedies. Wild mountain ginseng roots from the northern part of the United States, particularly in Wisconsin, Pennsylvania, and New York, are the most desirable, commercially favored products for exporting. These areas furnish roots of good size, weight, and shape, and they are generally considered the best breeding stock.[1] A related plant, the so-called dwarf ginseng, officially known as *Panax trifolium* Linn., is found from Nova Scotia to Wisconsin and Georgia. But this species is not desirable commercially.[2,3]

DISCOVERY OF AMERICAN GINSENG

A French Jesuit priest, Father P. Jartoux (1669-1720), with the help of P. Regis, serving as special topographic advisers to the Chinese Emperor Kanghsi, arrived in Peking in 1702. They were immediately sent to survey the remote lands in Manchuria, and on their journey they were able to visit the homeland of Chinese ginseng and experience first hand the healing power of ginseng. Father Jartoux was the first who furnished a detailed description of the Chinese ginseng *(P. ginseng)* plant in a letter that arrived in Paris on April 12, 1711.[2] The missionary described the plant as "a tartarian plant, called ginseng, with an account of its virtues in medicine. . ." In 1714 the missionary published the ginseng story in the *Philosophical Transaction* of the Royal Society of London. The news soon stimulated a serious interest in Europe in finding a miraculous panacea.

As a matter of fact, Chinese ginseng was not totally unknown to the Europeans, since back in the thirteenth century, Marco Polo, who found ginseng in general use throughout China, recorded it in his travel narrative in 1274 and made it known to other Europeans. He described the use of ginseng: "It was powdered, cooked, and used as a tea, syrup, or food condiment or even burned as incense in the sickroom. . ."[4] Later, Dutch merchants brought ginseng roots from the Orient to Europe in 1616, but except from some curiosity by the seamen no practical interest or attention was given it.

It was said that even the King of France who chose Chinese ginseng instead of several other very valuable gifts from Asia offered by a Siamese ambassador in Paris in 1686, since it was believed at that time that ginseng was the most precious panacea in the world. In 1697, the French Academy of Sciences conducted a discussion of ginseng, and ginseng in France was used for asthma, stomach disorders, and to promote fertility in women.[5]

Ginseng then became a desirable plant, and people in France turned to it with great enthusiasm. Michael Sarrasin, the king's physician for Canada, appointed by Louis XIV, collected some plants in Canada that were suspected of being ginseng plants.

The Indians in Canada knew about the ginseng plant, and they called it *Oteeragweh.* Some of the plants collected near Quebec by the Indians were sent to Paris for examination.[6,7]

Father Jartoux's communication did create a tremendous interest in the Western world, and suggested that the valuable root might be found in some countries, particularly French Canada where the forests and geographical environment are very close to those in Manchuria. Also fascinated about the ginseng business was a Jesuit missionary among the Iroquois Indians, Father Joseph Francis Lafitau, who also supposed that similar plants might be found in North America. After three months of laborious searching, Father Lafitau by accident did find plants that were very similar to what Father Jartoux had decribed. As a matter of fact, the color of the fruit of the plant attracted the attention of Father Lafitau, and this was responsible for the discovery of American ginseng near Montreal in 1716.[7]

In 1718, Dr. Sarrasin published in the *Memoirs* of the French Academy an account of American ginseng. Father Lafitau also reported his discovery of ginseng plants in the same year. Soon the big news reached Peking. Father Jartoux was very much interested in this big discovery and came to Canada to see the differences between American ginseng and its Chinese counterpart. Some ginseng roots were gathered and sent as samples to China for examination. Acknowledgement was slow in coming, but finally, the word arrived: "Your specimen lot is, indeed, ginseng; the quality is satisfactory. . . ." With this promise, soon the French began collecting ginseng, through Indians, for exporting. Soon the demand for ginseng thus created was so great that it became an important article of business in Montreal commerce.[8]

Before long, the short supply of wild ginseng in Canada became a serious problem. The ginseng trappers and traders spread the news of ginseng business to the American colonies. The American wildlife hunters thus became enthusiastic about not only furs but also ginseng roots. About thirty years after the discovery of ginseng in Canada, American ginseng plants were found in many parts of the northern American colonies. Ginseng was found in southern New England in 1750, and in central New York and in Massachusetts in 1751. It was similarly found plentiful in Vermont at the time of the settlement of the state.

Forest ginseng plants were eventually discovered in almost all states east of the Mississippi except in Florida, and in a few states west of the Mississippi River. It was growing wild in some parts of Maine, Connecticut, Rhode Island, Delaware, Pennsylvania, New Jersey, Maryland, Ohio, Virginia, West Virginia, Indiana, Illinois, Michigan, Iowa, Wisconsin, Minnesota, Kentucky, Tennessee, North and South Carolina, Georgia, Arkansas, and Alabama. A great part of the wild ginseng was found in those states touched by the Allegheny Mountains.

PANAX QUINQUEFOLIUM: GREEN GOLD

The American ginseng plant is a small, unassuming perennial herb, ten to twenty inches high. It is of very slow growth, even under the most favorable conditions. The plant is propagated from seeds, with stems bearing a single whorl of three palmately compound leaves, a solitary stalked umbel of greenish-white flowers, and bright red fruit. When the ginseng plant is old enough to produce fruit, it is rather noticeable and is easily recognized, but until three years old, it is not usually very prominent.

The seedlings at first somewhat resemble newly sprouted beans, in that they develop two cotyledons, and from between them a stem with two minute leaves. These enlarge until the plant has attained its first season's growth (about two inches). The growth of the plant during the first year is to develop the bud at the crown of the root, which is to produce the next season's stem and leaves. In autumn the stem dies and breaks off, leaving a scar, at the side of which is the solitary bud. In the spring of the second year, the bud produces a straight, erect stem, at the top of which one to three branch like stalks of the compound leaves appear. Three to eight leaflets are developed, which usually rise not more than four inches from the ground. The third year, eight to fifteen leaflets may be put forth, and the plant may attain a height of eight inches. In the succeeding years, the plant may produce three and five leafstalks three or four inches long, each bearing five thin leaflets

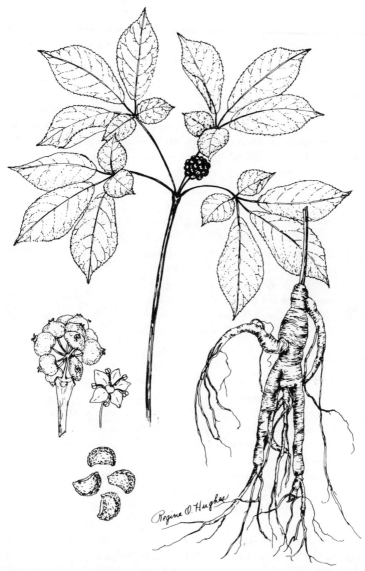

Branch, root, flower, berries, and seeds of American ginseng.

palmately arranged; two of them are smaller (an inch or two long), the remainder are larger (three or four inches), egg-shaped in outline, with the broad end away from the stem, abruptly pointed and raw-toothed. The leaves are bright green in summer, turing to yellow in the fall. The five-to-six-year-old plant grows from ten to fifteen inches in height from the ground.[1]

At the point where the leaf stalks meet, the main axis is continued into an erect but slender flower stalk, two to five inches long, bearing in early July or in late June a number of inconspicuous greenish-white flowers. These are soon followed by the fruit, which develops rapidly, remaining green until the middle of or late August, when it begins to turn sharp red, becoming scarlet and ripe in late September. The berries, which have the taste of the root, are the size and shape of small wax beans, and contain two or occasionally three seeds each.

No seed is produced in the first year, and only occasionally are berries found in the second year, and then only on extra-strong plants in the garden. It is only in the third year that the plant produces seed in any quantity. Plants in cultivated beds produce more freely than those in the forest. The largest stalk of wild ginseng seldom produces more than twenty or thirty seed berries, and only a few of these can be expected to survive and germinate, since many birds, mice, and chipmunks are very fond of ginseng seeds. On the other hand, the seeds must never be allowed to become completely dry or they may fail to germinate. In the forest, however, the seeds ripen in the autumn, fall to the ground, and are covered for eighteen months by the decayed leaves of the forest before the young seedlings appear. The seedlings must be properly protected and transplanted at least once before being set into the permanent beds. At all times, the beds must be kept free from weeds.

American ginseng usually has a thick, spindle-shaped root, two to three inches long or more, and about one-half to one inch in thickness, often branched, the outside prominently marked with circles or wrinkles. The root is simple at first, but after the second year it usually becomes forked or branched, and it is the branched root, especially, that vaguely resembles the arms and legs of a human body that used to be the particular favor in the eyes of the Chinese buyers. But this irrational belief is no longer held true. Ginseng has a thick, pale-yellowish white or brownish-yellow bark, prominently marked with transverse wrinkles, the whole root fleshy and somewhat flexible. If properly dried, it is solid and firm. It has a slight aromatic odor and the taste is slightly bitter followed by sweet and mucilageous. The dry root is about one-third the size of fresh ones. The best good-sized roots you find in the forest are from a few years to a few decades old. Though the roots acquire value from age, they do not increase much in size, five ounces (about 150 grams) being a giant root, but usually they are one to two ounces after dried. The dried root tastes slightly bitter and somewhat sweet afterward.[9]

The grading of ginseng roots is a highly subjective practice. The criteria are sources (wild or cultivated), shape, size, color (outside and inside), taste, texture, and markings. The trend has been toward continuously increasing in price since the beginning of the ginseng trade. A history of trade of American ginseng is given in the next chapter.

AMERICAN GINSENG ADVENTURE

In the state of nature, ginseng only propagates by seeds. If the plant is dug up prior to the ripening of the seed in September, it is deprived of its only means of perpetuating itself. Yet his was the very thing that happened to American ginseng. The *sang* diggers, a class of people that eked out a livelihood by hunting *sang* by shooting and trapping, exercised no judgement as to the season of digging. The plant was dug as soon as it was found in the forest, whether in April, May, or October. The other cause of the decreased supply of the wild root was the clearing of forest lands and the bruising and trampling of stock pastured in the woods. Both in Canada and in the United States, wild ginseng became extremely rare by the middle of the nineteenth century owing to extensive collecting without replacing. Nowadays the wild root is reported to have completely disappeared in many states where it used to be abundant. The ginseng plant seems to be extinguished entirely in Canada.

The visible decrease in the supply of the wild root and the constant increase in the demand as well as the increase in prices have led to many attempts at the cultivation of American ginseng by the *sang* diggers as early as in the early nineteenth century. But at that time failure was so frequent that its culture had once been declared impossible. However, such was not the case, since with proper attention and culture in an environment suited to its peculiarities, it may be grown successfully.

Until 1870, American ginseng was first successfully cultivated by Abraham Whisman at a place then called Boones Path in Virginia. Later George Stanton of Summit Station, New York, after long years of struggle succeeded to grow the plant in the 1880s. In the beginning he transplanted a few small wild seedlings and roots into his garden, and later he grew plants from the seeds of his own production. Not too long afterward, he became the first industrialized ginseng grower in the United States. He earned the title of "The Father of the American Ginseng Industry." In his eighty-square-foot "George Stanton's Chinese Ginseng Farm" in five years, he produced 320 pounds of ginseng root, which when dried, would have been about 106 pounds, harvested. The production was sold for $575, which was a sizable amount of income out of such a tiny garden. He was so devoted to his ginseng cultivation that he treated his plants as "babies," as he called them. It is more fascinating that Dr. A. R. Harding of Columbus, Ohio, began his cultivation of American ginseng in 1899. He gave up his regular medical practice and concentrated on ginseng experimentation. He had a wide observation along the lines of cultivation, propagation, and marketing of this valuable root in addition to its uses in the treatment of his patients. He transplanted and cultivated ginseng plants from each state and tested the extract in may types of patients. He believed ginseng was useful for many illnesses wherein regular treatment failed.

Between 1870 and 1895, there were about twenty ginseng gardens started. Ginseng farms mushroomed all over the

Eastern and Midwestern states during the so-called ginseng boom period between 1880 and 1903. However, a serious ginseng disease, Alternaria blight, broke out in 1904, caused a great damage to the crop, and hundreds of young ginseng farms were terminated. In the United States, only about six hundred acres of ginseng are planted. Ginseng farms in Georgia, Pennsylvania, but mainly in Wisconsin, are the principal cultivators. The average per-acre yield is about, 1,000 pounds and the total yearly harvest is from 100,000 to 150,000 pounds in the United States. The largest ginseng farm, the Framm Brothers of Hamburg, in western Wausau, Wisconsin, produces the most cultivated ginseng in the United States for domestic uses and exporting.

Part II

The Dollar Value
Of Ginseng And
Growing The Ginseng Plant

THE FLOURISHING GINSENG BUSINESS

AMERICAN GINSENG IN CHINESE MARKETS

Soon after the Chinese agreed to purchase American ginseng, a kind of ginseng stampede was ignited. Thousands of French Canadians and Indians took to the woods in quest of easy-to-dig "amber nuggets." A ginseng trading company was formed almost overnight. The rush for "green gold" was on. In Quebec the root was purchased at two francs a pound by the fur traders who collected and exported it to China. In China, the same root was sold for as much as twenty-five francs. Ginseng trade with China was at that time controlled by the Company of the Indies. In the beginning, the ginseng business was handled by the officers of the company. In 1751, seeing that the commerce in the root was so great, the company prohibited private venture on the part of its officers and assumed control itself. In only a short time the price of ginseng was advanced from twelve francs to thirty-three francs a pound.

Demands became so great that the *sang* (American ginseng) hunt became a highly profitable venture, particularly for the French Canadians. Exportation of the roots quickly increased; often the shrewd tradesmen unscrupulously received an average of ten to twelve times as much for *sang* as they paid uncomplaining diggers for it. The years rolled by, the tons upon tons of *sang* were ripped from Canadian soil. When finally demands could scarcely be met, many *sang* shipments started to yield inferior roots—roots were harvested out of season and improperly dried, leaving them visibly scorched.

In 1752 Chinese buyers inspected several shipments of American ginseng from Canada and found that the roots had been improperly treated and that a good portion of the roots were *not even ginseng*. This unprincipled practice all but ruined the Canadian *sang* market. Chinese traders were furious over the attempt to deceive them, and ginseng exports, in a year, dropped from over $100,000 to only $6,500. The ginseng trade in Canada thus dwindled rapidly and quietly faded away.[1]

The spark of demand for American ginseng was to remain dim for nearly thirty years, but gradually a limited and exceedingly wary market started once again to open its doors, and the favorable focus was on the American colony's ginseng roots. Ginseng grew naturally throughout the forest of most northern states, particularly the Appalachian Mountain areas, and the Chinese traders had confidence in the colonial roots — a stimulating business followed. Early American settlers often collected *sang* as a sideline and for a quick cash return. Local merchants accepted it in exchange for supplies, although fur buyers were the principal dealers.

The gathering and marketing of the root began in a small way, but picked up momentum when it was found that the range of the plant extended throughout the Eastern United States. Usually, the dry ginseng roots were purchased by the fur dealers in New York as well as other large cities. These buyers either disposed of their holdings to Chinese agents or exported directly to Hong Kong — the principal port of American goods entering China. There the roots were purchased in large quantities by the traders to supply the retailers or drugstores.

For many years, New York, Boston, and Philadelphia served as the main collection points for exporation of *sang*. The initial export from the United States to China started in the mid-eighteenth century, and the earliest trades were through the East India Company in England. A shipload of fifty-five tons of ginseng sailed from Boston to China in 1773. In 1782 the first direct shipment of American ginseng to China was made by John Jacob Astor. The root from that shipment was reported to have brought three dollars a pound. In Februrary 22, 1784, another American ship, *Empress of China* — a 360-ton ex-privateer—made another direct sail to China. Ginseng was the principal cargo. Daniel Boone, the great American pioneer and frontiersman, also collected and dealt in ginseng. In 1787 he started up the Ohio River with a fifteen-ton boatload of ginseng from Philadelphia on its way to China. Unexpectedly, he ran into trouble—the boat overturned.[2] Later the Chinese herbalists on the West Coast became the main ginseng dealers and exporters. During the end of the eighteenth century and beginning of the nineteenth century, American ginseng for export was mostly collected from the states of Pennsylvania, Ohio, Kentucky, and New York. A Kentucky buyer of ginseng noted that he had bought seventeen hundred pounds and he wanted to buy three hundred pounds more to make up a ton.[3] Such a large amount of dry root would bewilder a modern ginseng hunter and no doubt represented a collection acquired over an extended period, even then. In the 1790s, the wild root was selling for as high as one dollar a pound and about 200,000 pounds were exported each year to China.

The cultivation of transplanted ginseng seemed to have started some time in the 1840s. Due to the presence of the unnatural forestal ginseng in the shipment, the price was dropped from 68¢ in 1841 to 44¢ in 1842 and to 34 cents per pound in 1843. The Chinese buyers do not appreciate the cultivated species even though they are heavier and larger than the wild species. In 1858, about 366,053 pounds of ginseng, valued at $193,736, was exported to China. The price was fifty-two cents per pound. The export of *sang* continued through the years and the price continued to rise.

When the population moved westward, ginseng was discovered in abundance in the territory immediately west of Mississippi. About 1845, Green County of Wisconsin had acquired the reputation of being *sang* county.[4] Discovery of the American ginseng plant in many other counties followed, and by 1860 large amounts of Wisconsin wild ginseng were being collected and exported to China.[5] Later, ginseng collected in Minnesota was also exported to China.[6] The market price of ginseng in 1862 was then eighty cents and more a pound. By 1868 the market value of ginseng had doubled, and in that year, over 370,000 pounds of American ginseng reached

Chinese buyers. The price was even higher in 1878, and by 1888 it once again had doubled to two dollars and more a pound. But by now the inevitable was beginning to happen, and wild ginseng was becoming much more difficult to find. Even with the stimulation of higher prices, the year 1888 noted at least 112,000 pounds less than 1878; and in 1889 and 1890, with prices still higher, exported quantities took another sharp drop. In the year 1896, the price of wild ginseng climbed to $3.86 a pound, with only 199,000 pounds harvested. In 1897 only 179,573 pounds were exported, though the price jumped to the all-time high of $4.71, and the total value of ginseng exported to China reached $850,000. By the year 1898, the supply of wild ginseng became more scarce and many ginseng farmers began to harvest their cutivated product. Such extensive digging in quantity without even considering the age and without replacement contributed to the near extinction of the wild roots in the late nineteenth century.[1]

As a result of the scarcity of the wild root, the price rose up again to $5.20 a pound in 1900, $6.35 to $7.25 in 1907. The inflation was about five to ten percent per year. From that time on, more and more cultivated roots helped to fill the increasing demand from wild ginseng, which steadily became less and less available. Cultivated ginseng, tagged as such, was marketed and the price dropped once again from $4.70 to only $3.66 a pound.[7] However, due to the infinite demand for ginseng, soon the price jumped up to $7.00 again in the early twentieth century. The amount exported kept pace with the price, and the total export of *sang* exceeded one million dollars after 1905.

As a result of the attractive price, more and more people were involved. A ginseng boom took place in the United States in the years 1895 to 1904. Hundreds of new gardens were started, and stock companies were formed to grow and trade ginseng plants. Ginseng seeds were selling for about eight cents each or six dollars per ounce or ninety dollars per pound.[6] Unfortunately, a leaf disease of ginseng became prevalent in 1904, plaguing many plantations and discouraging the inexperienced growers.

Even during the First World War, the price of ginseng did not drop. By 1922, the market value of wild *sang* reached

$11.51 a pound, and top-grade large roots were bringing an even better price, while the cultivated roots were usually half the price of the wild species. The total exports valued more than two million dollars after 1922. The price of American ginseng remained high during the 1920s.

From the following tables, one can see that the demand for American ginseng has constantly increased since the trade started in the early eighteenth century, not only the export and total valuation but also the average price of American ginseng exported inflated from 1821 to 1975.[8]

Domestic Wholesale (Average) Price, Exports, and Total Value of American Ginseng from 1821 to 1920, Inclusive.

Year	Total Exported (lbs.)	Total Value	Average Price
1821	352,992	$ 171,786	$ .48
1822	753,717	313,943	.41
1823	385,877	150,976	.39
1824	600,046	229,080	.38
1825	475,974	144,599	.30
1841	640,967	437,245	.68
1842*	144,426	63,702	.44
1843	556,533	193,870	.34
1845	468,530	177,146	.37
1858	366,053	193,736	.52
1862	630,712	408,590	.84
1868	370,066	380,454	1.02
1878	421,395	497,247	1.13
1888	308,365	657,358	2.13
1889	271,228	634,091	2.33
1890	223,113	605,233	2.71
1892	228,916	803,529	3.51
1895	233,236	826,713	3.54
1897	179,573	846,686	4.71
1898	174,063	836,466	3.66
1900	160,101	833,710	5.20
1904	131,882	851,820	6.45
1905	146,576	1,069,849	7.30
1906	160,949	1,175,844	7.30
1908	154,180	1,111,994	7.21
1910	192,406	1,439,434	7.48
1912	155,308	1,119,301	7.20

1913	221,901	1,665,731	7.50
1914	224,605	1,832,686	8.15
1915	103,184	919,931	8.91
1916	256,082	1,597,508	6.23
1917	198,480	1,386,203	6.98
1918	259,892	1,717,548	6.60
1919	282,043	2,057,260	7.29
1920	160,050	1,875,384	11.71
1921	181,758	1,507,077	8.29

*The years in which cultivated ginseng was exported, mixed with wild ginseng, with a sharp drop in price.

Domestic Wholesale (Average) Price, Exports, and Total Value of American Ginseng from 1922 to 1975.

Year	Total Exported (lbs.)	Total Value	Average Price
1922	202,722	$ 2,334,918	$11.51
1923	148,385	2,245,258	15.13
1924	167,318	2,399,926	14.35
1925	138,131	1,668,221	12.07
1926	180,262	2,640,488	14.65
1927	169,000	2,556,000	15.12
1928	184,000	2,288,000	12.43
1929	234,000	2,766,000	11.82
1930	203,000	1,877,000	9.24
1931	265,000	1,922,000	7.25
1932	171,000	835,000	4.88
1933	233,400	844,000	8.62
1934	232,000	1,203,000	5.23
1935	167,000	618,000	3.70
1936	295,000	1,236,000	4.19
1937	136,000	706,000	5.18
1938	167,000	1,028,000	6.15
1964	139,206	2,731,602	19.62
1965	116,791	2,887,310	24.72
1966	173,405	4,358,542	25.13
1967	146,135	4,507,152	30.84
1968	133,701	4,359,524	32.61
1969	145,392	5,533,406	38.06
1970	162,689	5,016,951	30.83
1971	168,835	5,827,289	34.51
1972	227,549	8,922,426	39.21
1973	183,136	8,846,112	48.30

| 1974 | 216,832 | 11,116,787 | 51,27 |
| 1975* | 220,000 | 12,000,000 | 54.00 |

*Estimated.

During the Sino-Japanese War and the World War II years, there was little American ginseng exported to China, although the amount did reach 185,976 pounds in 1946; a downward trend appeared in 1947 and later years. But the demand for American ginseng began to increase after 1950, and also most of the ginseng was exported to Hong Kong instead of to China. In 1951, the market value of American ginseng in Hong Kong was about $17.57 a pound, and some unusual roots were valued at more than $130 per pound.[9]

Since 1964, the demand for American ginseng once again has increased constantly. As is shown in the preceding table more than two million dollars worth of ginseng was exported from the United States after 1964, with increases reaching four million dollars in 1966, five million dollars in 1969, and eight million dollars in 1972. As a result of Richard Nixon's visit to China in 1972, American ginseng sales suddenly boomed in Hong Kong. China takes all the ginseng that American growers and ginseng hunters can supply. In 1973, of the total export of American ginseng valued at about nine million dollars, the Chinese buyers in Hong Kong took about ninety four percent of the total supply. Similarly in 1974, the total American ginseng exported was about $11.1 million, and about twelve million dollars in 1975.[10] The current wholesale prices are about fifty dollars to sixty dollars per pound for wild ginseng, and about thirty dollars to forty dollars per pound for cultivated American ginseng at New York City's fur traders. The price fluctuates tremendously due to the sources, the age, and the quality of the root. Even as it is today, the wild ginseng roots are much more highly priced than the cultivated roots, because they grow naturally. All of the American ginseng exporting records were kept at the Bureau of Census of the U.S. Department of Commerce.

The United States will experience stiff competition for the ginseng market in the Orient from now on. Both Japan and South Korea, and perhaps later, China, are big ginseng growers and suppliers in Hong Kong at lower prices for better ginseng roots. In 1973 the United States price hit nearly fifty dollars per pound, compared to Japan's twenty-five dollars and South Korea's thirty-five dollars per pound.[11]

A STORY OF AMERICAN GINSENG HUNTING

Ginseng hunters and trappers frequently carried digging tools, food, etc., and went into the woods to hunt for the "green gold," and sometimes even women and boys hunted the roots. The plant was well known to all mountain children, and few were the mountain cabins that had no ginseng in them waiting for market.

Albert Burnworth, the veteran ginseng digger, who lived near Ohiopyle, Fayette County of Pennsylvania, recalls the days of his memorable "sang'n" (ginseng hunting). The following passages are quoted from his own words published in the *Pennsylvania Anguler:*[1]

Most people who know the stuff and who have dug it call it "sang" — and that includes me.

In front of his shaded porch, he said:

Almost everywhere hereabout "sang" was beginning to show the effect of over-digging when I was a boy. But there were some nice patches to be found from time to time. I had no idea what the Chinese people did with "sang". I just knew that it could buy the things that people needed. In many families both girls and boys learned early to distinguish "sang" from other woods plants. Taken to a local country storekeeper the roots could be exchanged for school clothes and household needs. Shipped to the big buyers it brought money that made dreams come true. Many a boy got his first fishing tackle and his first gun and pocket watch with "sang" money.

Asked if he could think of just one old-timer who had done a great deal of sang digging, Mr. Burnworth replied:

Not one. They are all gone, almost like the "sang" is gone. But there were some good "sang" diggers in this locality. This rich

Youghiogheny watershed produced some big old "sang" roots; but personally I can't tell of digging any extremely large roots, the biggest being just a fraction under half a pound, and it ws shaped like a parsnip. I reckon maybe the tales of some "sang" roots are like a few of the stories about big fish — stretched a bit. And that reminds me, that it wasn't uncommon for "sang" diggers of my day to get in some fishing while on a root-hunting jaunt. In fact I had line and hooks with me a good part of the time when I was "sanging". I have dug hundreds of pounds of "sang" and always found the north slopes best suited to its growth. "Sang" likes cold weather and high elevations and it almost never freezes out. I usually aimed to do most of my "sanging" in the fall when the "sang" berries were ripe; and all that I found I'd plant in hard-to-get-to places along the slopes of steep hollows and the like.

He continued:

I think that "sang" was struck the biggest blow during the Great Depression Years. A lot of country people scoured the hills for it and in a way, you couldn't blame them. A pound of dry "sang" would buy a nice lot of groceries for a hungry family, or pay a doctor or buy lots of clothes; and two pounds would buy a good cow. But it's sad to think of wild "sang" being just about a thing of the past. Scarcity always does wild things to prices, and I guess that's why "sang" is now fetching about forty-two dollars a pound. I know of a couple of nice stalks of wild "sang" in a hard-to-find nook. Some of my memories make them almost sacred, so for now, I guess their whereabouts will have to be my secret. . . .

THE FLOURISHING KOREAN GINSENG BUSINESS

Korea earned its fame and prestige as the ginseng country. The favorable soil and climate, particularly in the mountain areas, have provided ideal conditions for producing the highest quality Korean ginseng roots. In the past two thousand years, ginseng has been one of the biggest sources of income to the Korean government and its people. From 1896 to 1901, Korea exported about 7,000 *catties* of white ginseng, and about 30,000 to 90,000 *catties* of red ginseng to China each year. The price for white ginseng was 76 yen while for red ginseng, 2,183 yen per *catty*.[12] Before the Second World War, Korea exported about 26,000 *catties* of red ginseng to China each year, which earned more than \$1.2 million.[13] After the World War II, the Korean government continued to keep the monopoly system to manage the ginseng business. The Office of Monopoly was established in Seoul to cultivate, manufacture, and ex-

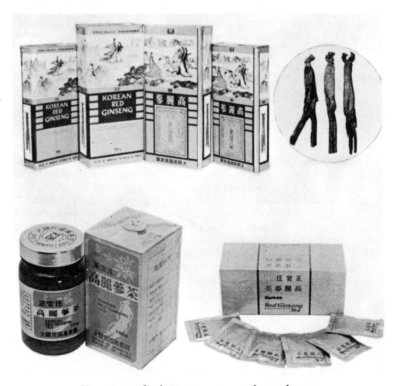

Korean red ginseng roots and products.

port, Korean red ginseng products. On the other hand, many privately owned ginseng farms were then born to cultivate ginseng plants making white ginseng products. As a result of systematic and industrialized cultivation in recent years, ginseng harvestation and exportation had significant growth.

South Korea has become the number one ginseng grower and exporter in the world.[14]

Korean ginseng root used for exportation have a wide variety of specifications, i.e., size, color, and age, and are sometimes quite puzzling to the buyers. Two kinds of ginseng roots are most common for export: the red ginseng and white ginseng roots. There are at least six grades or classes of Korean red ginseng roots.[14] According to the Korean government's export standard, the red ginseng are:

Heaven Brand. . . . . First Class
Earth Brand. . . . . Second Class
Good Brand. . . . . Third Class
Large Tails. . . . . Fourth Class
Small Tails. . . . . Fifth Class
Cut Brand. . . . . Sixth Class

The current price for first-class Korean red ginseng is about $200 per 600 grams retail at Chinatown, New York's drugstores.

The Korean white ginseng roots are usually doubly cheaper than the red ones. Similarly, the classification is based on the age, size, and weight of the root.[14] Evidently, there are six grades of white ginseng roots, which are:

Per 600 gram box contains:
Class A. . . . . No more thatn 10 roots
Class B. . . . . Not less than 11, but not more than 20 roots
Class C. . . . . Not less than 21, but not more than 30 roots
Class D. . . . . Not less than 31, but not more than 40 roots
Class E. . . . . Not less than 41, but not more than 50 roots
Class F. . . . . More than 50 roots

The Class A white root is currently sold at about fifty dollars to sixty dollars, and the Class E grade white root is sold at about thirty-six dollars per six hundred grams, F.O.B. Korean port.

Korean red ginseng is famed throughout the world for being the highest quality, and the only competitors for international markets come from China and North Korea. The United States, Canada, and Japan are keen competitors in the sale of white ginseng root. However, since the Office of Monopoly guaranteed the quality of ginseng roots and their processed products, the exportation of red ginseng alone reached to $9.6 million in 1973, from $5.3 million in 1972, with a growth of about eighty-two percent in one year. Exportation of white

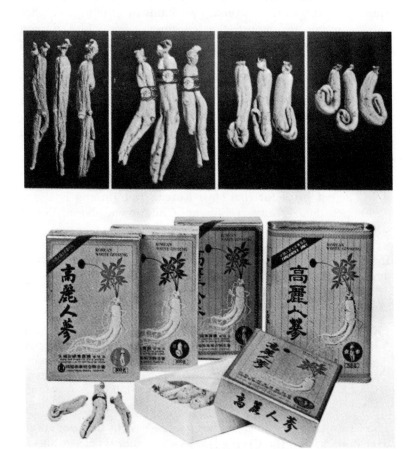

Korean white ginseng roots.

ginseng and its products is similarly subject to government inspection. In 1970, Japan imported more than two million dollars worth of Korean white ginseng. The biggest customers of white ginseng next to Japan are West Germany and Switzerland. They usually import the top-grade white ginseng, while Japan, on the other hand, prefers the lower grade or the cheapest roots.

Currently, Korean ginseng products are shipped abroad by about thirty major ginseng industrial firms. Red ginseng is primarily exported to Hong Kong, followed by the United States, Singapore, the Federal Republic of Germany, Japan, Thailand, France, Italy, Holland, Canada, South American, and African countries. Korean white ginseng products are mostly shipped to Japan, Hong Kong, Switzerland, West Germany, Malaya, and the Middle East countries, according to the Office of Monopoly.

In addition to red ginseng and white ginseng roots, exported items also include ginseng in syrup or "honey ginseng," instant ginseng tea, ginseng cake and candy, ginseng extract, ginseng powder, ginseng drink, ginseng tablets, ginseng capsules, ginseng pills, ginseng fluid extract, ginseng tincture, ginseng elixir, ginseng wine, and ginseng electuary. Most of the above products have been found only recently in health food stores and Oriental drugstores in the United States.

In the last ten years, the Korean ginseng business has had records of fantastic growth. According to the Office of Monopoly, in 1970 the total amount of ginseng products exported was $8.3 million in comparison with $3.7 million in 1968, and only $492,000 in 1963. In the last five years, the growth has been even bigger. It earned about $14.2 million in 1972, $23 million in 1973, and $31 million in 1974, and is expected to reach a $45 million target in 1975 of total exportation of Korean ginseng products. In the last ten years, each year had about thirty percent to fifty percent net growth, which indicates that ginseng is indeed selling very well. If the ginseng-loving population could be doubled in the next two to three years, one would expect Korean ginseng exportation to double, and the $100 million target would not be difficult to reach.

THE GINSENG BUSINESS IN JAPAN

The market value of the crude cultivated *Panax ginseng* in Japan varies considerably with the sources of production and age. The Fukushima ginseng root is the cheapest, the Nagano ginseng root is medium priced, and the Shimane ginseng root is the most expensive. For example, in 1973, the six-year-old Fukushima root was sold at 3,500 yen, Nagano root was sold at 4,500 yen, and Shimane root was sold at 6,000 yen per kg. From 1970 to 1973, prices went up at rate of about ten percent to twenty percent each year as are shown in the following table. Accordingly, the Japanese ginseng root was sold in Japan at about $6.17 in 1970, $6.21 in 1971, $6.80 in 1972, and $7.05 per pound in 1973. The price of a five-year-old root is cheaper than a six-year-old root by about ten percent to fifteen percent, while a four-year-old root is cheaper than a five-year-old root by another ten percent.

Annual Exportation of Red Ginseng, White Ginseng, and
Other Ginseng Products from Japan

Y e a r		Red Ginseng	White Ginseng	Others	Total*
1970 Kg.		80,984	4,633	2,051	
	1000¥	1,251,260	54,038	14,152	1,319,450 ($4,398,166)
1971 Kg.		110,416	4,219	47,815	
	1000¥	1,875,346	49,551	12,462	1,937,359 ($6,457,(863)
1972 Kg.		88,185	4,094	4,537	
	1000¥	1,352,126	41,235	25,987	1,419,342 ($4,731,140)
1973 Kg.		83,764	3,529	11,390	
	1000¥	1,360,572	39,436	133,596	1,534,104 ($5,113,680)
1974 Kg.		109,376	4,142	13,980	
	1000¥	2,695,058	49,936	163,414	2,908,408 ($9,694,693)

*According to the current rate of 1 U.S. $= 300¥.

The annual production of cultivated ginseng in Japan is about 319,000 kg (or 703,200 lbs.) including four, five, and six-year-old roots. Based on the market value of the different roots, the total value of Japanese ginseng is about $4.3 million.

The best ginseng roots are usually made into red ginseng for exportation. The inferior roots are made into white ginseng and other processed ginseng products consumed domestically or exported. The processed ginseng products are ginseng extract, ginseng tincture, tea, etc., sold at heathfood stores.

Japanese ginseng exportation is similarly a very flourishing business. In 1970, Japan exported ginseng products valued at about $4.4 million, $6.4 million in 1971, $4.7 million in 1972, $5.1 million in 1973, $9.7 million in 1974, and $10 million in 1975. Nearly ninety-five percent of the products are exported to Hong Kong, and the rest of the products are exported to Singapore, Thailand, West Germany, France and the United States.[15]

CURRENT REGULATION OF GINSENG PRODUCTS

In the last few years, the import of foreign ginseng and ginseng products has become a boom. Almost all healthfood stores, Oriental-goods stores, and even some American drugstores are now stocked with and selling imported ginseng products from Korea, the USSR and China. Ginseng tea, extracts, tablets, and capsules have been best sellers. These products are sold as food, not as drugs.

Because modern scientific information on the medicinal value of ginseng has not reached the hands of government agencies, ginseng is still banned from being marketed domestically as a drug. The Bureau of Drugs of the Food and Drug Administration (FDA) has been effectively prohibiting the importation and marketing in the United States of all forms of pharmaeceutical ginseng products bearing medical claims. The Bureau of Foods of the FDA similarly issued a guidance several years ago that: "We are not aware of any evidence tending to establish that ginseng should be generally recognized safe for use in alcoholic beverage or as flavoring agent in carbonated beverages or soft drinks." The Bureau of

Foods, however, permits the import and marketing of ginseng roots and other ginseng products provided that no nutritional or therapeutic claims are made on the labels of the products.[16]

THE GINSENG DEALERS

In the last few years, a new booming ginseng business became prevalent. Herb shops, almost all healthfood stores, Oriental-goods stores, and even drugstores are now selling foreign as well as American ginseng products. You have no problem in getting all kinds of modern ginseng products in almost all large cities in the United States and many countries in Europe. While it is impractical to provide a complete list of ginseng dealers in the United States, the firms listed in the following are a few dealers selling modern ginseng products, with the understanding that no discrimination is intended and no guarantee of reliability implied. The market prices of these ginseng products, as you may have already found out, vary significantly as a result of sources, brand, packaging, strength, etc. It is a good idea to write or visit several different firms or stores finding out which store you think is most reasonable. Also, to shop wisely, you may call or send for their catalogs and prices. Since ginseng products are sold over the counter or by mail orders, no prescription is needed.

Ginseng Roots and Ginseng Products Sellers

Eastern States

Chuen Hing Co.
215 East 26th Street
New York, N. Y.
(212) MU 6-5013

Gae Poong Korean Ginseng
40-15 150th Street
Flushing, New York, N.Y.
(212) 539-6366)

Tung Yen Tong Co.
19 Pell Street
New York, N. Y. 10013
(212) 233-9586

Tong Fl Enterprises, Inc.
99-17 Queens Blvd.
Flushing, N.Y., N.Y.
(212) 459-1666

Kiehl Pharmacy
109 3rd Avenue
New York, N.Y.
(212) 475 3400

Herb Society of America
300 Massachusetts Avenue
Boston, Mass.
(617) 536-7136

Haussmann's Pharmacy
6th and Girard Avenue
Phila., Pa.
(215) MA7-7707

Penn Herb Co.
603 N. 2nd Street
Phila., Pa.
(215) WA5-3336

The Seed
3420 Sansom Street
Phila., Pa.
(215) EV2-7554

We and Me Herb Tonic Co.
261 S. 60th Street
Phila., Pa.
(215) SH8-3230

Chinese American Trading Co.
91 Mulberry Street
New York, N.Y. 10013
(212) CO7-5224

Wah Yin Hong Enterprises, Inc.
81 Mott Street
New York, N.Y. 10013
(212) 964-4290

Sphinx Self Exploration Book
Store and Herb Shop
948 Massachusetts Avenue
Boston, Mass.
(617) 491-8788

American Horse Inc.
119 Meyran Avenue
Pittsburgh, Pa.
(412) 687-1500

Kinley Drug Store
7401 Frankstown
Pittsburgh, Pa.
(412) 731-3804

Central States

Botanical Medicine Co.
10601 W. Warren Ave.
Detroit, Mich.
(313) 581-9190

Europe Import Co.
13525 Gratiot St.
Detroit, Mich.
(313) LA7-2425

Merco Herbalist
620 Wyandotte E. Windsor
Ontario
(519) 253-9472

P. C. Jezewski Drugs
10042 Jos Camp Ham
Detroit, Mich.
(313) TR2-5898

Natural Life Health Foods
207½ W. McMillan
Cincinnati, Ohio
(513) 651 — 5288

Western States

Nature's Herb Co.
281 Ellis Street
San Francisco, Calif.
(415) 474-2756

Superior Trading Co.
837 Washington Street
San Francisco, Calif. 94108
(415) 982-8722

The Lhasa Karnak Herb Co.
2482 Telegraph Ave.
Berkeley, Calif.
(415) 548-0380

Bing's Tailoring and Import Co.
1280A Green Street
San Francisco, Calif.
(415) 776-4496

Star Herb Co.
38 Miller Ave.
Mill Valley, Calif.
(415) 383-3318

Umbrella Herb Co.
831 Almar, SCR, Calif.
(408) 423-7913

Herbal Life Products
12926 Saticoy NH, Calif.
(213) 765-5433

Chientan and Co.
1030 S. Alvarado
Los Angeles, Calif.
(213) 388-2769

The Herb Lady
Box 26515
Los Angeles, Calif. 90026
(213) 666-8480

Herb Products
11012 Magnolia
N. Hollywood, Calif.
(213) 877-9220

The Fmali Co.
831 Almer Ave.
Santa Cruz, Calif. 95061
(408) 423-7913

Many fur dealers in New York and other large cities also are American ginseng root buyers and sellers. The market price of American ginseng fluctuates more or less, chiefly because of trade conditions and the demand. The following firms deal primarily in American ginseng, American ginseng seeds and seedlings. While it is impractical to provide a complete and up-to-date list of American ginseng dealers in the United States, the firms and individuals provided here, it is believed, are active in business. However, in a changing world, conditions can change overnight to affect almost everyone's business. Contact several of these firms to see which vendor suits you best. I make no claims as to the honesty or integrity of any of the following dealers.

American Ginseng Root Growers or Dealers

Eastern States

United Fur Brokers
258 West 29th Street
New York, N. Y. 10001

H. R. Hutt
RFD #1
Oswegatchie, N. Y. 13670

Coeburn Produce Co.
Lacy E. Fuller
Coeburn, Va. 24230

F. Amco Lt.
844 St. Martin Dr.
P. P. Box 5142
Va. Beach, Va. 23455

James F. Farmer Co.
Lebanon, Va. 24266

Robert Group
RD #2
Gardners, Pa. 17324

Wm. J. Boehner and Co.
259 West 30th Street
New York, N. Y. 10001
(211) 695-3435

Geo. E. Warren
South Schroon
New York, N.Y. 12877

Broadwater Trading Co.
Jim Broadwater
Cate City, Va. 24251

V. H. Holmes and Son
959 Big Creek Rd.
Richlands, Va. 24641

Lakeland Nurseries Sales
Hanover, Pa. 17331

Central States

W. C. Peters
Antigo, Wis. 54409

Heise's Wausau Farms
Route 2
Wausau, Wis. 54401

Elmwood Ginseng Gardens
2329 12th Street
Akron, Ohio 44314

Mifflin Fur Co.
Ashland, Ohio 44805

F. B. Collins
Box 126
Viola, Iowa 52350

Black Forest Botanicals
Box 34F.
Yuba, Wis. 54672

Fromm Brothers, Inc.
Route 1
Hamburg, Wis. 54438

T. U. Hardacre
Route 1
Wadsworth, Ohio 44281

The Gurney Seed and Nursery Co.
Yankton, S. D. 57078

C. Wade
Rm. 613
Indianapolis, Ind. 46204

Indiana Botanical Co.
P. O. Box 5
Hammond, Ind. 46325

Southern States

Smoky Mountain Drug Co.
Arthur Slaughter
935 Shelby Street
Bristol, Tenn. 37620

Wilcox Drug Co.
Kenneth Wilcox
Boone, N.C. 28607

Blue Ridge Drug Co.
West Jefferson, N.C.

S.B. Penick and Co.
Asheville, N.C.

Q. C. Plott and Ginseng Co.
4062 Peachtree Rd.
Atlanta, Ga. 30319

Stills Ginseng Mountain
214 NA 33 Echodale Lane
Knoxville, Tenn. 37920

Ginseng
Box 4F475
Flagpole, Tenn. 37657

Ginseng Gardens
Ashville, N.C. 28801

Greer Drug and Chemical Corp.
Lenoir, N.C.

Todd Harb Co.
West Jefferson, N.C.

Vol Braschears
Combs, Arkansas, 72721

7
GROWING YOUR OWN GINSENG PLANT

It has been fully demonstrated that ginseng plants can be raised successfully in a field where the necessary conditions are furnished. That is to say, the ginseng plants must be provided
with a forestlike environment.[1,2,3,4] Those who own forest lands
can grow ginseng plants easily. Also, it was formerly thought
that ginseng could grow only under conditions exclusive to the
Far East. However, experimental work has shown that ginseng
can be raised successfully in many parts of the north temperate
zone: in some regions of European Russia and of southeastern
Europe, in eastern Siberia, and in North America.[5] Ginseng
can be grown from seeds, seedlings, or roots. Plants free from
blight or mildew and growing spontaneously in the woodland
can be transplanted to prepared gardens. Ginseng is a very
slow-growing and an exacting crop. It will be disappointing if
not properly managed.

The cultivation of ginseng, since the beginning, has been a
promising and profitable industry. As a crop, however, ginseng
is no gold mine, but it certainly gives a reasonable return to
growers who are willing to care for the crop for at least the five
or six years that are required to reach maturity. The total
acreage of ginseng farms in the whole world today is not sufficient to meet the demand of the market. Should there be a
temporary decline in price, or should a glut occur, as
sometimes been the case, a grower need lose nothing, since he
may leave the roots in the ground for one year or more, know-
ing that they are improving in size and quality. Other advan-
tages of the ginseng industry are that it may be started and

continued without excessive outlay, and may be confined to land that otherwise could not be used for cultivated crops. When properly cultivated, a very small area may be made to yield a very large proportionate return.

Ginseng has become an increasingly important medicinal plant in the Western world since World War II. To meet the demand, improvement in methods of ginseng cultivation and control of typical ginseng diseases have been attained through extensive agricultural research in the Orient, the United States, and the Soviet Union. At the present, increasing cultivation and output are the main concerns of ginseng-producing countries.[6]

It is most probable that the demand for ginseng will increase in the foreseeable future. The price will, naturally, continue to go up and up. This has been the case for the last two hundred years. The large-scale industrialized cultivation of *P. ginseng* in China, Korea, Japan, and perhaps Siberia would certainly affect the market for American ginseng. Nevertheless, the world market for ginseng has been so great that it far exceeds the supply. With more and more people turning to ginseng, the demand could double in the next decade. If you are a potential ginseng grower, you need not worry about the market.

CULTIVATION OF GINSENG IN THE ORIENT

Growing ginseng is a rather difficult job because it does not grow in conditions different from its natural environment. Ginseng grows most happily in the northern temperate zone between 36^0 and 38^0 north, where the degree of humidity is exactly suited to its prima donna temperament. At all stages in its development, the young ginseng plant must be protected from snow, rain, frost, hurricane, and, most important of all, direct sunlight. The plant is covered with thatched shades like terraced rows of little bus shelters. The ginseng plant, by nature, is a dark lover, growing without the need of too much sunshine or radiant energy. Accordingly, receiving the right amount of light is important during its growth.

The root is not harvested until it has reached the sixth year, and by that time it has sucked nearly all the natural nutrients from the earth that the field cannot be reused for another ginseng crop for about ten to fifteen years. Top-quality soil produces superior ginseng. For the seedbed, a soil of sand or gravelly sand formed through weathering of granite, gneiss, and calcite is recommended. For the field, soils composed of a texture of sandy clay loam, sandy loam, and loamy sand are suitable. All types of chemical fertilizers are found unsatisfactory or even harmful for growing ginseng plants. Special composites, called *yakto,* are used to increase the high quality of the root. The *yakto* is a complex product made from fermenting the raw foliage of broad-leaved trees and a small amount of green grass, cotton-seed cake, soybean cake, and defatted rice bran. Fermented human waste mixed with animal waste, tree ashes, and chimney soot have also been used. In both the seedbed and the field, *yakto* or natural fertilizer is usually employed as the prime source of nutrient. The first-grade bed soil is made with sufficient *yakto* and chimney soot. The nutrients absorbed by the plant thus stimulate its growth. The quality of the ginseng root, no doubt, depends upon the soil and nutrients used during cultivation.

Seeds are taken from four-year-old plants and raised to seedling stage in carefully drained seedbeds. The season for sowing seeds of ginseng is preferably in late October or early November. The seeds grow in a nursery for one and a half years, and in March or April they are transplanted into the field or permanent beds. Usually, the seedlings are planted out in beds raised a foot above the level of the surrounding soil, bordered with upright slates and covered from heavy sun and rain by shades of reeds three or four feet high, well closed in, except toward the north side, where they are left more or less open, according to the weather.

Sheds are placed in rows with just enough room to walk between them. Ginseng is transplanted frequently during this period. Ginseng rarely blooms in less than two years, older plants start flowering around the middle of May and bear red fruit in middle or late July. The stem is about six inches high with four horizontal leaves standing out from the stem at right

angles, and in the fifth year, a strong, healthy plant has reached maturity, though it is usual not to take it up until it has
reached the sixth year. The roots, after harvesting in autumn,
are very carefully washed and scraped, and are then treated in
one of two ways traditionally used by the Chinese (see chapter
2), yielding white or red ginseng roots, respectively.

The ginseng seed has a hard coat on its surface, and since
the embryo is incomplete, some manipulation is necessary for
accelerating its germination. Methods to accelerate germination, the control of typical ginseng plant diseases, and the interrelation between the raising process and the environment
have been under intensive research in the Orient. The results
of these types of studies are covered in the following sections.

GROWING GINSENG IN THE UNITED STATES

Ginseng grows naturally on slopes of ravines and in well-
drained sites where soil is formed from acid leaf mold of hardwood forests. The soil should be naturally dry and fairly light,
and in condition to grow good vegetables without the addition
of strong manure. By proper treatment almost any fairly good
soil can be conditioned for ginseng growing. The addition of
woodland soil tends to produce hard, flinty roots of inferior
quality.

In the book called *Ginseng and Other Medicinal Plants,*
written by A. R. Harding in 1908, detailed information on the
habits and cultivation of American ginseng is given.[4] The
Farmer's Bulletin, Nos. 1184 and 2201, published by U.S.
Department of Agriculture, also give detailed information on
growing American ginseng. The following information on
growing and harvesting American ginseng given in this chapter
is based on the *Farmer's Bulletin,* Nos. 1184 and 2201, respectively.

First of all, American ginseng must be provided with
favorable conditions for growth. Selection of the proper loca-
tion, preparation of the soil, and good drainage are important
in planting ginseng. The best site for beds is a hardwood forest,

with tall trees to provide favorable dense shade, and with little
undergrowth. Similar drainage and shade conditions should be
maintained when growing ginseng in lath sheds. Make beds
four feet wide with walkways between them. For root planting
work the beds up to twelve inches deep. For seeds and seedlings, work the beds only eight inches or so deep to prevent set-
tling. Mound the center of permanent planting beds to provide
space for more plants and, if located on flat ground, to
facilitate good runoff of water. Slope the walkways so that they
will drain water from the beds during heavy rains. The most
favorable conditions for the soil are a rich, sandy, loamy soil.
Clay land can be used, but one has to mix it with leaf mold,
rotten wood and leaves, and some light soil, and it must be
thoroughly pulverized.

Ginseng needs three-fourths shade during the summer and
free circulation of air. The proper amount of shade can be provided in lath sheds or by trees in a forest planting. Laths should
run north to south to provide alternating sun and shade to the
plant. Do not use burlap or muslin; they interfere with air circulation.

For seedbeds, break up soil to a depth of six to eight inches,
and remove all weeds, grasses, and roots. Mix one-to-one with
fiber-free woodland soil. If the soil is inclined to be heavy, add
enough sand so that mixture will not harden after heavy rain.

Use of seeds instead of seedlings may prevent the introduc-
tion of disease to new plantations. Also, this is the least expensive way to start a plantation, but requires a longer period until
harvest.

Seeds ripen in the fall, but generally do not germinate until
the following fall. Do not allow ripe seeds to dry out. Store
them in a cool, moist place. Use woodland soil, sand, loam, or
sawdust as a storage medium.

Plant seeds in the spring, as soon as the soil can be tilled.
Only scarified or partially germinated seeds should be used for
planting. They are planted eight inches apart each way in permanent beds, or two by six inches apart in seedbeds. Cover
seeds with one inch of forest soil, or well-rotted or basswood
sawdust; do not use pine or oak sawdust.

Some growers plant the seeds when they ripen in September, and cover the beds with leaf mold or mulch. They keep the beds covered until spring, when the seeds begin to sprout.

Ginseng seedlings are more expensive than seeds, but a crop grown from seedlings can be harvested two or three years sooner than a crop propagated from seeds. Several firms sell one-, two- or three-year-old seedlings. Three-year-old seedlings produce seed during the first fall after planting, which may be used for planting future crops. Set seedlings in permanent beds, eight inches apart each way. Closer spacing tends to increase disease in the plantation.

Roots may be set any time from October to April, after the soil has been tilled. Fall planting, however, is usually preferred. Plant roots two inches below the bed surface, and eight inches apart each way. When roots are not available from woodlands, beginners should purchase them from reputable growers. Roots grow more rapidly when not permitted to seed.

Ginseng may be grown directly in woodlots, or in lath sheds with partial shade — an environment similar to the plant's natural habitat. Plants thrive best in loamy soil, such as found in oak and sugar maple forests in the North. Shade is essential.

Ginseng requires relatively little cultivation. The beds should be kept free of grass and weeds, and the soil should be scratched with a light implement whenever it shows signs of caking. One active man can easily take care of about two acres of ginseng.

A winter mulch over the crown is essential to prevent heaving by frost. A four- or five-inch layer is ample in the most severe climate; less is needed in the South. Spread mulch when frost is imminent and remove it in the spring before the first shoots appear. Light mulching to retain moisture during dry weather is also advisable. Forest leaves or light brush, held in place with poultry netting, makes the best mulch. Cornstalks stripped of husks, bean vines, cowpea hay, and buckwheat straw are also suitable if they do not contain weeds, seeds, or other materials attractive to rodents.

Many growers are opposed to excessive use of fertilizers. Heavy use of barnyard and chemical fertilizers lessens the resemblance of cultivated ginseng to the wild root. Over-manuring also forces growth and lowers the resistance of ginseng to the attack of disease.

Some growers fertilize with leaves or old sawdust from hardwood trees, or with ground-up, rotten hardwood. Others prefer woodland soil or rotted leaves four to six inches deep, spaded to a depth of about eight inches, with fine, raw bonemeal well worked in, and applied at the rate of one pound per square yard.

Fence beds to keep out animals and to discourage theft. Protect the beds from moles with boards or close-mesh wire netting set twelve to eighteen inches in the ground. Rodents may be controlled with traps.

A ginseng crop matures in five to seven years. Generally the roots are dug in mid-October of the sixth year. Good roots are about four inches long, one inch thick below the crown, and average one ounce in the fresh state. Older roots possess the most substance and when properly cured bring the hightest prices.

The proper time for digging ginseng roots is in autumn, mostly in October, and they should be carefully washed, sorted, and slowly dried. If the ginseng roots are collected at other seasons of the year, they will shrink more and not have the fine, plump appearance of the fall-dug root. Dig the roots with their forks intact. Carefully free them of adhering soil so as to preserve their natural color and characteristic circular markings. Do not scrape or scrub them. The market value of the product is based, in part, on wholeness and appearance. Some growers replant young and undersized roots, or heel them in until spring planting.

The clean, fresh roots are usually dried in a well-ventilated heated room, at about 60-80° F. and after a few days, the temperature of the room can be raised up to 90° F. until the roots dry. Spread the roots thinly on lattice or wire-netting shelves. Turn them frequently but handle with care to avoid marring the surface or breaking the small branches. Roots more than two inches in diameter will need to be dried for about six weeks. During damp and very wet weather, care should be taken to see that the roots do not mold or sour. They should never be overheated, since this will tend to discolor the surface and spoil the texture of the roots. Too fast drying at too high a temperature damages the roots both physically and chemically. When all cured, the roots should be stored in a dry, airy, and rodent-proof place or in containers.

It is of great importance that the roots should be properly treated for marketing. They should never be split in washing or drying. The little neck or bud-stem should be unbroken, for if it is missing, the roots lose two-thirds of their value in the market. In the ginseng business, as in other trades, there are tricks. The tricky ginseng diggers have been known to try to adulterate the ginseng shipments with pokeweed and other roots. The inexperienced buyer may at times be fooled, but not the dealer who really knows his business. Ginseng roots have also been doctored with thin slivers of lead and other weights to make them heavier. Sometimes, depending on how skillfully the insert is made and camouflaged, the deceptive scheme is difficult to detect. Of course artificial weight has to be added when the ginseng is green, and sometimes the drying process cracks the roots and exposes the petty fraud! No matter how well it grades out, Chinese buyers never rate American ginseng better than *third* class.

The cultivation of American ginseng and the control of ginseng diseases have been researched by both governmental agencies and many Agriculture Experiment Stations at state colleges and universities during the ginseng boom years. In 1895, the U.S. Department of Agriculture published *Farmers Bulletin* (No. 16) entitled "American Ginseng, Its Commercial History, Protection, and Cultivation." The request for this bulletin was great enough to require the revision and printing of a new edition in 1898. In 1902, the bulletin was again reprinted with the addition of a "Note of Warning" signed by Frederick V. Coville calling attention to a "BOOM" in the sale of ginseng seeds and roots. Because of the extravagant prices, fraudulent and adulterated species were unavoidable. In 1904 and after, bulletins on ginseng culture and diseases were also published by state agricultural experiment stations in Pennsylvania, New York, Kentucky, Missouri, and possibly elsewhere. In 1913, a new ginseng bulletin (No. 551) written by V. F. Valter, entitled "The Cultivation of American Ginseng" was published. In 1921, the U.S. Department of Agriculture issued another bulletin, *Farmer's Bulletin* No. 1184, edited by W. W. Stockberger, entitled "Ginseng Culture" and reprinted in 1941 and 1953. The most recent issue of a ginseng bulletin, the *Farmer's Bulletin* No. 2201, written by L. Williams, entitled "Growing Ginseng" was issued in 1963. The requests were so enormous that the same bulletin had to be reprinted in 1964 and 1973.

We do not know how many Americans are still interested in growing ginseng plants today, but there are many. A recent article in the *New York Times*[5] described how Denver Davis grows his ginseng plants in the hills of northern Georgia. Mr. Davis started growing ginseng as a hobby nineteen years ago. He said: "When I first started, the first year I got a matchbox full of seeds, and I thought I had done some good. Now I am digging 12 bushels a year, getting two gallons of seeds." On his two-acre ginseng farm, the ginseng plants are from one to fifteen years old, and most of them are mature and ready to harvest. Once the plants are mature, the tops are discarded, the roots harvested, and dried in a heated building like a tobacco barn. They lose two-thirds of their weight in moisture before the pale-yellow roots are ready for sale. Another ginseng grower, Mr. Gooch, also of Georgia, owns a four-acre ginseng farm. He harvests three hundred to six hundred pounds of ginseng root per acre worth twenty dollars to thirty dollars a pound to dealers, while the dealers, usually fur and hide traders, sell at as high as sixty dollars a pound to the Asian buyers. Talking about growing your own ginseng plant, Mr. Davis said: "You have to week it five to six times a year, the moles and rats are after it all the time. A lazy man ain't going to grow it."

SPEEDING UP GERMINATION AND GROWTH

Since in the newly ripened seeds the embryo is not yet formed, the sprouting of ginseng seeds usually takes about eighteen to twenty-two months. The development of the embryo, under natural conditions, takes several additional months after ripening of the seeds. This fact was revealed only a few years ago, but the Chinese and Korean ginseng growers long empirically knew about this and worked out special methods of pre-sowing treatment of the seeds. However, their traditional methods proved not be satisfactory according to the standard of modern agriculture.[6]

Seeds stratified immediately upon ripening sprouted after eight months; those stratified after four months of storage under dry conditions sprouted in nineteen months. In the last few years, Japanese and Soviet botanists have developed a new and effective method of hastening germination with a chemical agent called gibberellic acid.[6] Gibberellic acid has been widely used in promoting growth of plants, especially the growth of seedlings.[7] Gibberellic acid belongs to the family Giberellins, and so far at least fourteen gibberellins have been isolated. This plant growth promoter is obtained from the fungus *Gibberella fujikoroi* (Sawada) Wollenweber.

The Soviet botanists Grushvitskii and Limari found that in the ginseng seeds treated with gibberellic acid, the length of the first stage of after-ripening is reduced from four to two months; consequently, the whole period of preparation of the seeds for sowing is reduced from eight to six months.[8] According to Japanese agriculturalists Ohsumi and Miyazawa, when ginseng seeds were soaked in various concentrations of gibberellic acid solution and incubated in a sand bed, gibberellin promoted the growth of the embryo and, as a result, raised the rate of germination.[9] The germinating power, or the number of seeds germinated, was increased approximately from 50%-70% to 90%-100%. The best results were obtained if the seeds were previously treated with 0.05% to 0.1% of gibberellic acid solution over a period of twenty five hours.[10]

Other germination-promoting agents, such as kinetin, naphthal-epeacetic acid, indole-3-acetic acid, 2,4-D in addition to gibberellic acid were also tested. The best growth-promoting agent, so far detected, was gibberellic acid. Recent studies in Japan used a 100 p.p.m. aqueous solution of gibberellic acid in which seeds were immersed for twenty-four hours, and germination of seeds was accelerated by lowering the temperature to 2^0-15^0C. for about ten days. The optimum temperature for germination was found to be 10^0C.[11]

The effect of light intensity and of pH of the culture medium on ginseng plant growth has been reported recently by T. Kuribayashi and associates.[12,13] Two-year-old plants were grown in Wagner sand pots and supplied with Hoogland and Arnon nurient solution. The light intensity was adjusted to 100%, 50%, 30%, 10%, and 5% of natural normal sunlight, and the pH of the soil was adjusted to 3, 4, 5, 6, 7, and 8, respectively. After four months of cultivation, it was found that no plant survived at the 100% and 50% light intensity, whereas the majority of the plants survived at 5%-10% sunlight (about 3,000 to 6,000 lux.) intensity. High alkalinity destroys ginseng plants. Many ginseng plants died at the environment soil of pH 7 and 8, whereas they grow normally in pH 4, 5, and 6 medium. Accordingly, 5%-10% sunlight intensity, and the slightly acidic environment medium with pH of 5 to 6 are the most optimum conditions for ginseng growing.[14]

Research also indicates that light has a significant effect on the absorption of the nutrient by the plant. The concentration of the plant nitrogen, phosphur, and potassium are different under different light intensity conditions. The maximum rate of intake of these nutritive substances by the plant is under shade or dark conditions. The common forest soil on which ginseng normally thrives is usually brownish-gray in color containing relatively greater amount of aluminum, calcium, magnesium, nitrogen, organic matters, and sulfur. Plant research shows that soil with a relatively higher content of sulfur, magnesium, calcium, in addition to the other three essential nutrients, is very important for promoting the normal growth of ginseng culture.

PART III

The Truth
About The Manroot

8

GINSENG INFORMATION AND
SCIENTIFIC RESEARCH

THE UNPOPULAR PANACEA

The age-old panacea tonic is not popular in the Western countries at all, particularly in United States. At the present time, little modern scientific information about ginseng is available, and the majority of the people, even health-care professionals, know little about ginseng.

Recently, I inquired of thirty-three information librarians at twenty-four good-sized public and drug-companys' libraries in the New York metropolitan area about ginseng. "Ginseng? I never heard of it." After searching their filing cards and reference books they said, "Sorry, we don't have any of the latest scientific information about ginseng." Twenty-six librarians gave me the same answer. Seven librarians, however, told me: "Ginseng, it is an Oriental tonic. It gives you power and vitality." Two among them not only knew about ginseng but they told me that they are currently using it. Regardless, no single library could provide me with any scientific references. Instead they showed me some obsolete legends and tales about ginseng found in several booklets or encyclopedias about medical plants and herbs.

From 1971 to 1976, only three out of ten larger newspaper publishers printed articles on ginseng. *The New York Times* published three articles: "Ginseng — Seoul's Oldest Export" appeared on March 14, 1971;[1] "Bars Sale of Sex Stimulant" appeared on April 25, 1972;[2] and "Ginseng Root Is a Minor Cash Crop for Georgians" appeared on October 11, 1975.[3] The *Wall Street Journal* reported an article: "Lowly Ginseng Plant Is One Root to Profit for Some Americans," appearing on September 9, 1975.[4] The *Milwaukee Journal* reported two articles: "Interest in Growing Ginseng Root Renewed," and "Ginseng Still has a Lot of People Rooting For It," appearing on April 8, 1973 and December 13, 1974, respectively.[5,6] The other seven newspapers I surveyed (e.g., *Examiner of San Francisco, Chicago's Tribune*, the *Philadelphia Inquirer, Star of Montreal, Star Telegram of Fort Worth, Los Angeles' Herald Examiner*, and *Register of New Haven*) had no record of printing any article related to ginseng.

Modern German, French, and Anglo-American standard textbooks of medicinal chemistry, pharmacology, and therapeutics, and other medical reference books do not contain ginseng in their index. Textbooks of pharmacognosy are the only professional books that provide information on ginseng. One pharmacognosy book says: "Ginseng is a stimulant and a stomachic. It is a favorite remedy in Chinese medicine."[7] Another pharmacognosy book states: "Ginseng contains glycoside called Panaquilon, panax sapoginol, volatile oil, a physosterin, mucilage, a sugar, starch, etc. Ginseng is used by the laity as a stimulant and aromatic bitter. The Chinese employ it as an aphrodisiac and heart tonic but without scientific identification."[8] A third pharmacognosy book, which is the newest one, refers to ginseng: "Ginseng is a favorite remedy in Chinese medicine and is considered to have tonic, stimulant, diuretic, and carminative properties. It reportedly reduces the blood sugar concentration and acts favorably on metabolism, the central nervous system, and on endocrine secretion. It is employed in the Orient in the treatment of anemia, diabetes, insomnia, neurasthenia, gastritis, and especially, sexual impotence. . . ."[9]

American ginseng remained on the official *United States Pharmacopeia* (USP)[10] list of acceptable herb drugs from 1842 to 1882 but only as a supplementary drug for stomachic and stimulant uses. During the first half of the twentieth century, ginseng was officially listed as demulcent in the *United States*

Dispensatory (USD)[11] and *National Formulary* (NF)[12], as well as USP. However, ginseng was dismissed as a therapeutically useless drug and was deleted from the official compendia in 1950; that was the end of American ginseng and since then, nobody wants to talk about it. For about twenty-five years, ginseng has been unknown to the majority of the American public.

THE GAP OF SCIENTIFIC INFORMATION

There has been a serious problem in finding scientific information on ginseng in the Western countries, since nearly all ginseng research work has been conducted in the Orient and in the Soviet Union and published in their native languages of Chinese, Korean, Japanese, and Russian, in difficult-to-obtain or obscure journals. No library in the Western countries, including the Library of Congress and the National Library of Medicine, has a complete collection of foreign journals.

The *Index Medicus*[13] does not list as many ginseng articles as did the *Chemical Abstract*.[14] I made a complete survey and found about three hundred pieces of ginseng information listed in the entire *Chemical Abstract* starting with the first volume of 1907 up to Volume 84 of the current year. By no means is it a complete collection, for it is impossible for the Chemical Abstract Service to collect and translate all of the foreign papers of every discipline. The *Chemical Abstract* is not easily accessible to the American public.

American professional journals have not published any ginseng articles in the last twenty-five years, since few studies on ginseng were conducted in the United States. Questions often are raised nowadays by many customers to their pharmacists, by patients, many retired people, and some business-minded ginseng enthusiasts who want to grow ginseng or formulate ginseng for products, yet not one single booklet that is currently available tells the modern scientific findings about ginseng. A letter from the Agricultural Research Center of the U.S. Department of Agriculture written to me said, "Although the Department does not conduct research studies on ginseng, every year we receive thousands of request for information on its culture, marketing and uses. . . .[15] Another correspondent also from the Agricultural Research Service Center at Beltsville, Maryland, wrote to me: "With the increased interest in acupuncture, I note an increased interest in Oriental medicinal plants. I get more inquiries about ginseng than about any other medicinal plant."[16] The American public is desperately searching for new evidence about ginseng.

MODERN SCIENTIFIC RESEARCH AND PUBLICATIONS

The earliest chemical and pharmacological studies on ginseng started in the mid-ninteenth century. As a matter of fact, it was started right here in the United States with the American ginseng root collected in Canada. The first chemical report was published in 1854.[17] At that time it was extremely difficult to obtain any large quantity of authentic specimens of American wild ginseng, and also due to the extravagant prices, studies were limited and little fruitful results were made before 1900.

After the turn of the twentieth century, most of the preliminary studies were conducted by the Japanese. From 1900 to 1935, ginseng studies became one of the most active projects at many pharmaceutical colleges and medical centers. As a result of the annex of Korea by the Japanese military and later their occupation of Manchuria, the Japanese then possessed all the valuable roots, as they had desperately desired for centuries. Within thirty-five years time, about fifty studies were conducted in the areas of chemical, biochemical, pharmacological, and even clinical trials on ginseng extracts — not only ginseng from Manchuria and Korea, but also specimens of American ginseng. Although their results did not reach a clear conclusion that ginseng is useful for treatment of certain ailments, their results stimulated the interest of scientists in Western countries including the USSR.

From 1936 to 1945, ginseng research was interrupted as a result of the Sino-Japanese War (1937-45) and World War II

(1939-45). Few ginseng scientific papers are seen in the literature published between 1936 and 1950.

Being the next-door neighbor to China, the Russians, following the track of Japanese, showed tremendous interest in Chinese ginseng. As early as in 1859, a scientific expedition was organized in St. Petersburg (now Leningrad) to explore the Manchu territory and the frontier of Korea and examine especially the ginseng and other Chinese plantations with a view of establishing plantations on Russian soil for the purpose of trade with China.[18]

Prior to the Second World War, limited studies on ginseng were conducted at the Institute of Experimental Medicine of the USSR. During 1945 and 1948, the Red Army invaded Korea and Manchuria, thus the ginseng-rich lands were then transferred from Japanese to the Russians. Supposedly the Red Army then grabbed the entire supply of ginseng valued at about $120 million, and shipped it to home for studies and consumption. A special institution called The Institute of Biologically Active Substances, Siberia Department of Academy of Sciences of the USSR, was soon established in Vladivostok in 1949. The function of the newly established organization was to conduct research on medicinally useful herbs found in China and Siberia, particularly ginseng. The Vladivostok center coordinates all related pharmacological, clinical, and chemical investigations from Vladivostok, Novosibirsk, Khabarovsk, Leningrad, Tomak, Moscow, and many other cities of the USSR. In 1965, this institute moved into an excellently equipped new laboratory building erected on the picturesque shore of the Armur Ray. A special ginseng committee uniting the efforts of all scientists and clinicians engaged in this field has been working since 1949. Up to 1965, the committee held twenty-three sessions in which not only Soviet but foreign scientists participated as well. The committee has issued seven volumes of works and a two-volume collection of the minutes of the committee sessions.[19] Through extensive research, the Soviet scientists, in collaboration with the Japanese, have established the nature, the structure, and the medicinal properties of the active principles of ginseng.

In South Korea, as well as in China, ginseng research work, mostly confined to the pharmacological and physiological aspects, was started after 1956. New methods of growing and of controlling typical ginseng diseases were also explored. Little chemical work however, was published, as is true today.

Since 1960, a new era of ginseng research was started. As a result of the availability of modern instrumentation and technique, in addition to an ardent interest in ginseng research in Asia and some parts of Europe, significant accomplishments have been made.

In the last fifteen years, at least 160 chemical papers have been published. Dr. Elyakov and his associates at Vladivostok and Professor S. Shibata and his co-workers at the Faculty of Pharmaceutical Sciences, University of Tokyo, are the outstanding scientists who have successfully isolated and identified the ginseng saponins from *Panax ginseng* root as well as from other species. Scientists who have similarly contributed significantly toward the understanding of ginseng chemistry are: Professor Horhammer of the University of Munich; Professor Kondo of the School of Pharmaceutical Sciences, Showa Univiersity, who has established the structures of chemical constituents of Japanese ginseng; and Professor Staba of the College of Pharmacy, University of Minnesota, whom with his co-workers, has been studying extensively the American ginseng plant and the mechanism of biosynthesis of ginseng saponins.

The biological studies of ginseng from 1930 to 1960 by Japanese workers, the Soviet scientists at Vladivostok, and by Bulgarian, Chinese, and South Korean scholars, they all used crude ginseng extracts, either aqueous or alcoholic, as the testing materials. Researchers began to evaluate the activities of ginseng by using the purified saponins as testing material, or the different fractions of extraction since 1970. This is, no doubt, the beginning of a new milestone in ginseng research. Thus, the biological data on ginseng's activities, using chemically purified material and identified specimens, are much more scientifically meaningful and valid. Much remains to be done, however, in the study of the biomedical and biochemical actions of ginseng and its clinical trials must still be conducted.

Ginseng Symposium The first international ginseng symposium, sponsored by the Central Research Institute of the Korean Office of Monopoly, convened in Seoul in September 1974.[20] Some five hundred well-known scientists, pressmen, businessmen, and government officials from Belgium, Britain, Japan, Singapore, Sweden, South Korea, Switzerland, Taiwan, Thailand, the Netherlands, Turkey, and the United States, and West Germany attended the meeting. The ginseng scientists and ginseng enthusiasts sat together to discuss the different aspects of ginseng, its pharmacology, composition, clinical aspects, and modern methods of cultivation.

The meeting opened with a keynote speech by the president of the symposium, Choi, Yoon-kuk, director of the Central Research Institute of the Office of Monopoly. "The symposium is designed to provide an opportunity for international exchange of academic and scientific information concerning ginseng," Choi said. Lee, Chang-suk, the vice-minister of the Ministry of Science and Technology, echoed the same theme with a reminder that "Research on the properties of ginseng is proceeding both in the Occident and the Orient."

Regarding the pharmacological properties of ginseng, research papers were given by, respectively, Professor K. Takagi of the University of Tokyo; Professor Hong, Sa-ak of the College of Medicine, Seoul National University; Dr. Ivan Popvov of the Renaissance Revitalization Center at Nassau, Bahamas; Professor Dr. Finn Sandberg of the University of Upsala, Sweden; Dr. Karl Reuckert, managing director of Pharmaton, Ltd. in Switzerland; and Dr. Lee, Kwang-soo, of the State University of New York. In addition, a review of information on ginseng pharmacological work was presented by Prof. Karlfried Karzel of the University of Bonn.

In the areas of chemical composition and biochemical effect of ginseng, papers were presented by Professor Dr. L. Horhammer of Munchen University; Dr. S. Shibata of Tokyo University; Professor S. Hiai of Toyama University; Professor M. Yamamoto of Osaka University; and Dr. John Staba of the University of Minnesota.

On the cultivation of ginseng, Professor Lee, Choon-young, of Suwon Agriculture College reported his study of the chemical quality of the nursery and soil of ginseng cultivation. Professor Yeng, Young-tu, of the Taiwan Agricultural Institute reported the effect of various mulching cultivations on ginseng root and quality. Dr. Changyawl Harn of the Korea Atomic Energy Research Institute reported his study of the systematic cultivation of ginseng.

The second international ginseng symposium, sponsored by Pharmaton Ltd. and the World Health Organization, convened on April 9 to 12, 1975, in Lugano, Switzerland.[21] Similarly, the objective of the meeting was to discuss scientific research and exchange ideas on ginseng.

In the total 122 years history of ginseng's research, about 750 scientific articles have been published altogether by a few hundred scientists in twelve countries. Among these papers, seventy percent are biological studies, twenty percent are chemical, and the rest are botanical and reviews. The current interests are the broad clinical trials and the chemical synthesis of the ginseng saponin structure out of economical sources. Finding ginseng substitutes is another project scientists are seriously undertaking with keen interest.

9
SECRET PRINCIPLES OF GINSENG

The Bible says that for every disease there is an herb in the plant kingdom. The plant kingdom provides a tremendous reservoir of natural crude drugs. In the past thousands of years, people of all over the world, particularly the Chinese, have consumed considerable quantities of botanical drugs, more frequently called herbal drugs. Like energy and minerals, the herbals remain the primary source of supply of many clinically useful remedies.

The virtue of the herbal remedies is that most of these natural products have proved to be medicinally effective, mild, and relatively safe. *Ma Huang*, described as a remedy for coughs and as a cardiac stimulant, is one of the oldest Chinese herbals. Liquorice root has been used in medicine for treating stomach complaints and as a general sweetner in China as well as in other countries for many centuries. A third example, the snakeroot *(Rauwalfia cerpentina)*, has been used by the Indians as a tranquilizer for more than four hundred decades.

How do ancient herbals become modern medicine? It is true that a great number of modern remedies used in the United States are from a natural source. You must have used or at least heard of ephedra, ergot, digitalis, penicillin, codeine, morphine, cocaine, quinine, atropine, and hundreds of others derived from nature. To obtain therapeutically useful principles from the crude herbs, as a rule, the medicinally useful or biologically active principles are isolated by suitable extractions, separations, and purifications. The important principles contained in the crude drugs are called *constituents*. Some of the constituents may be biologically active, while others may be inert, thus medicinally valueless. The most commonly encountered principles such as cellulose, lignin, suberin, cutin, starch, and coloring matter are inert materials, whereas glycosides, alkaloids, vitamins, enzymes, volatile oils, fixed oils, and acids are important biologically active constituents. In the old days, the crude water extractions or decoctions of drugs were frequently used in the treatment of diseases. In modern times, however, the crude extracts are usually further processed to obtain purified principles. In order to find out how good the herbal drug, its extract, or its purified materials are, pharmacological and toxicological studies are carried out with laboratory animals. With promising animal evidence, preliminary clinical trials in humans may be conducted. Efficacy and long-term toxicity studies are the last steps in developing a new drug. To develop a new chemical drug, drug companies usually spend an average of five to ten years and more than $12,000,000 from its synthesis to marketing. The development of drugs out of natural sources, the cost may be even higher.

We recall that soon after the isolation of reserpine from the snakeroot, it became the most important tranquilizer in the treatment of hypertension. Another example is aspirin. After the discovery of salicin in the bark of willow trees, it has been developed as the most versatile, and most widely prescribed drug in history. Even in modern times, since the discovery of penicillin in 1929, thousands of new penicillins have been prepared and a great many have been used clinically.

Among the five botanically identified *Panax* species *(Panax ginseng, P. quinquefolium, P. trifolium, P. japonicum, P. pseudoginseng,* except *P. trifolium,* all have been used as crude drugs in the Orient. Although Siberia ginseng *(Eleutherococcus senticosus)* does not belong to the genus *Panax,* it possesses similar medicinal activities as does ginseng. All these plants are botanically related, i.e., they all belong to the family Araliaceae. These plants do not, howver, contain the same active constituents, nor do they possess the same medicinal values. The kinds of chemical principles contained in the various *Panax* or ginseng plants are the subject to be discussed in this chapter.

CHEMICAL RESEARCH ON *PANAX GINSENG*

In the course of chemical studies on ginseng, chemist have attempted to isolate and identify ginseng's active principles, and thus verify the usefulness of ginseng.

Rafinesque seemed to be the first who reported his findings of a camphorlike substance, Panacene, from an extract of American ginseng root in 1854.[1] Almost simultaneously, Garriques also reported his findings that, from a crude extract of American ginseng root, he obtained a yellowish glycoside called Panaquilon.[2] Panaquilon is soluble in water and alcohol, but insoluble in ether. Its sweet taste resembles that of licorice root. After acid hydrolysis, panaquilon gives a water-insoluble substance called Panacon. Later in 1889, a Soviet worker, Davydow, reported that he similarly obtained a ginseng glycoside from extracts of Manchurian ginseng roots, and its properties were similar to panaguilon.[3]

Pioneer studies were also conducted by quite a number of Japanese chemists during the 1900s. Inoue isolated a substance from an extract of Japanese ginseng *(chikusetsu ninjin).*[4] This substance was shown to be a saponin glycoside. It has some hemolytic (breaking down of red blood cells) properties. In 1905, Fujitani isolated a relatively pure saponin from the extracts of Korean and Japanese ginseng roots.[5] It was a white crystalline powder and was similarly called panaquilon. In the following year, Asahina and Taguchi reported that from an alcoholic extract of ginseng root, a noncrystalline substance was obtained.[6]

More detailed chemical studies on ginseng were conducted by Dr. Kondo and his associates. The powdered ginseng roots were extracted with water, methanol, and ether, respectively. A mucilageous substance and some inorganic substances were found in the aqueous extract; a mixture containing cane sugar, nitrogenous substances, and a saponin glycoside was obtained from the methanol extract; and oily substance, brown in color with typical ginseng fragrance, was obtained from the ether extract. The ginseng oil was further fractionated with steam distillation into two portions, i.e., a light yellowish volatile oil, and a brown, nonvolatile portion. The volatile oil contained panacene, while the nonvolatile fraction was shown to contain phytosterol and fatty acids. Upon hydrolysis of the saponin glycoside with seven percent alcoholic-hydrochloric acid, two new substances, panax-sapogenol and panax-sapogenol-amorphous (noncrystalline), were obtained. Further studies showed that the ginseng saponin glycoside consisted of one mole of panax-sapogenol, two moles of glucose, and one mole of pentose, and the molecular weight of the saponin glycoside was 876. From quite a number of authentic samples, it was found that the cultivated Korean and Japanese ginseng gave similar chemical components.[7,8,9] Abe and Saito[10] and Yonekawa[11] together isolated a relatively pure ginseng saponin glycoside, ginsenin, from Korean ginseng root. Pharmacological studies were conducted with ginsenin. In 1930, Kotake similarly isolated a ginseng saponin which was called panaxin, but this substance did not show haemolytic properties. After hydrolysis of panaxin with fifty percent sufuric acid in methanol, a new substance, α-panaxin was obtained. α-panaxin was the sapogenin (aglycone) of ginseng extract.[12] α-panaxin was further degradated with fuming hydrochloric acid, giving glucose and a halogenated compound called aglucone. Sakai, on the other hand, had more interest in the fragrant ginseng oil. From an ether extract of ginseng roots, a considerable amount of sweet-smelling, and biologically active ginseng oil was obtained. The most active component of the oils that represents the activities of the whole ginseng was the volatile oil portion called panacene. The ether extract also contained a number of other ingredients. High molecular weight unsaturated fatty acids, called panax acids, and esters of fatty acids have been isolated.[13,14,15,16]

In the last sixteen years, great advancement has been made in isolation, characterization, and identification of the principles of ginseng, and ginseng saponin chemistry, first in history, has become known to the scientific world.

By using different solvent systems, it was found that some of the ginseng constituents are only extractable with water or alcohols, while others are primarily organic solvent or oily soluble. The crude extracts have been successfully separated with the aid of thin-layer chromatography (TLC) and column chromatography techniques. The TLC has been a very useful tool that separates ginseng saponins of very similar structures. Infra-red (IR), NMR, and mass spectroscopy, on the other hand, have provided the powerful means for elucidating the structures of the useful principles contained in the mysterious root.

Based on the chemical studies of ginseng, we now learned that *Panax ginseng* root contain, quite a number of biologically active and medicinally useful components.[17,18,19] According to their chemical nature, these numerous components, so far identified, can be classified into nine groups:

- ginseng saponins (saponin glycosides)
- ginseng oil and phytosterol
- sugars and carbohydrates
- organic acids
- nonprotein nitrogenous substances
- amino acids and peptides
- vitamins
- minerals and trace elements
- unknown enzymes

It has been confirmed pharmacologically that the chief biologically active components in ginseng and other *Panax* species appear to be ginseng saponins. Ginseng roots contain a substantial amount of ginseng saponins; accordingly, it is the saponins that contribute most, if not all, of the important pharmacological activities of ginseng extract. The chemical properties of these important ginseng principles will be discussed further in the following sections.

GINSENG SAPONINS

Saponins, a sweet-bitter material, usually exist in plant in the form of glycosides known as "saponin glycosides." Ginseng, sarsaparilla, glycyrrhiza, etc. contain a considerable amount of saponin glycosides. Saponin glycosides are giant molecules that are extractable from the plant materials by hot water or alcohols. Saponins have particular chemical properties, and the most notable characteristics are: (1) forming colloidal solutions in water that foam upon shaking (frothing); (2) having a bitter taste; (3) having sternutatory and irritating properties to the mucous membrane; and (4) having hemolytic action against red blood cells.[20,21]

Composition and Physical Properties of Ginseng Saponin Glycosides
Panaxosides Isolated from *P. Ginseng* C. A. Mey.

Panaxoside	Melting Point, t°C.	Molecular Weight	Composition	
			Genin (sapogenin) +	sugar (mol)
A	176-8°	—	panaxatriol	glucose (3)
B	182-5°	—	panaxatriol	glucose (2) + rhamnose (1)
C	185-7°	1031-1064	panaxatriol	glucose (3) + rhamnose (1)
D	157-60°	1178	panaxadiol	glucose (4)
E	185-7°	1222-1230	panaxadiol	glucose (4) + arabinose (1)
F	185-7°	1388-1424	panaxadiol	glucose (6)

A number of ginseng saponin glycosides have been isolated from the methanol extracts of ginseng roots and identified by the Soviet workers at Vladivostok and Moscow. These saponins are called panaxosides.[22,23] In 1962 Elyakov et al., reported that they were successful in isolating saponin glycosides, panaxosides A and B.[24] Two years later, four additional saponins, panaxosides C, D, E, and F, were isolated.[25] Based on composition, these six ginseng saponin glycosides belong to two groups. Panaxosides A, B, and C belong to one group and they yield a common nonsugar substance (aglycone) called panaxatriol, while panaxosides D, E, and F belong to another group and yield panaxadiol after acid hydrolysis. None of the six panaxosides carries identical sugars. Panaxoside A consists of three glucoses; panaxoside B, two glocoses, and one rhamnose; panaxoside C, three glucoses and one rhamnose; panaxoside D, four glocoses; panaxoside E, four glocoses and one arabinose; panaxoside F, six glucoses.[25,26] The composition and some of the physical properties of panaxosides are listed in the previous table. In 1974, Andreev *et al.* were able to isolate a total of fourteen spots on the TLC plates, each spot representing one different ginseng glycoside or panaxoside.[27] In cooperation with the Japanese workers, the structures and the properties of these panaxosides have been identified.

In 1962, Professors Funjita, Itokawa, and Shibata of the University of Tokyo, were able to isolate two types of compounds, saponin glycosides and sapogenin (aglycones), from the methanol extracts of three different species of ginseng roots (ginseng, Japanese ginseng, and American ginseng).[28] The ginseng saponin glycosides isolated by the Japanese workers were called ginsenosides, which is quite different from the Soviet nomenclature (panaxosides). Sapogenins (the nonsugar portion of saponin glycoside) are normally obtained when the saponin glycosides are treated with hot hydrochloric acid (HCl) in methanol. Soon it was learned that the sapogenins thus obtained were not true sapogenins but actually the acid hydrolyzed products of ginseng saponins. Soon the structure of the acid hydrolyzed saponin was identified as panaxadiol.[29,30,31] Immediately Dr. Shibata's group was successful in confirming that the structure of panaxadiol is a tetracyclic, triterpene of dammarane structure.[31,32]

The genuine sapogenin of ginseng was eventually obtained when the ginseng extracts or the saponins were hydrolyzed under mild conditions (0.7 percent sulfuric acid) in methanol solution. The true sapogenin, thus obtained, was called prosapogenin,[33] and the chemical structure of it was identified as protopanaxadiol.[34]

After a series of comparative studies, it is confirmed that panaquilon (originally isolated by Garriques), panaxin (isolated by Kotake), and ginsenin (isolated by Yonekawa), are the same saponin. Panacon (isolated by Garriques, α-panaxin (isolated by Kotake in 1930), and a compound that melted at temperatures greater than 270°C. obtained by Asahina *et al.* are identical with prosapogenin, the so-called genuine aglycone of ginseng, which melts at 330°C.[28]

In 1965, more than ten neutral ginseng saponins were isolated by the thin-layer chromatographic technique and they were designated as ginsenoside Rx (where x = a, b, c, d, e, f, g-1, g-2, g-3 and h). Hydrolysis of ginsenosides R_b and R_c, panaxadiol, was obtained. Similarly, hydrolysis of ginsenoside Rg-1, however, a new sapogenin, panaxatriol, was isolated. All physicochemical data indicate that panaxatriol is a homologue of panaxadiol and carries one more OH group than panaxadiol.[35]

Shibata *et al.* in 1974 successfully isolated thirteen ginsenosides from ginseng root extract. They are: R_o, R_a, R_{b_1}, R_{b_2}, R_c, R_d, R_e, R_f, R_{g_1}, R_{g_2}, R_{g_3}, R_{h_1}, and R_{h_2}. The ginsenosides from R_o to R_h correlate the increased R_f value of the TLC. Ginsenoside R_o is the least polar, having the lowest R_f value. From the TLC plates, ginsenosides R_{b_1} and R_{b_2} (R_b group) and R_{g_1}, R_{g_2}, and R_{g_3}, (R_g group) are noted to be the main components of the saponins.[36]

The detailed compositions or structures of these saponins were not known until 1968, when Professors Iida, Tanaka, and Shibata reported that the composition of ginsenoside $R_{g\text{-}1}$ is composed of protopanaxatriol and two glucose molecules. At present, nine of the total thirteen ginsenosides have been characterized, and their structures have been established.[36,37,38] The physical form, melting point, chemical formula, and characteristic IR of the nine ginsenosides are listed in the following table.

According to the nonsugar portion of the molecule, these ginsenosides can be divided into three groups. Ginsenoside R_o gives oleanolic acid (aglycone), while ginsenosides R_b, R_c, and R_d give panaxadiol, and ginsenosides R_e, R_f, and R_g give panaxatriol after acid hydrolysis. Ginsenoside R_o is quite a different compound in comparison with other ginseng saponins, but it is identical to chikusetsu saponin V, a saponin isolated from Japanese ginseng.

Physical Properties of Ginsenosides

Ginsenosides	Physical Properties	Melting Point (t°C)	Formula	IR (KBr) cm^{-1}
R_o	Colorless needles (MeOH)	239-41	$C_{48}H_{76}O_{19}$	3400 (OH) 1740 (COOR) 1728 (COOH)
R_{b_1}	White Powder EtOH-BuOH)	197-98	$C_{54}H_{92}O_{23}$	3400 (OH) 1620 (C=C)
R_{b_2}	White Powder EtOH-BuOH)	200-3	$C_{53}H_{90}O_{22}$	3400 (OH) 1620 (C=C)
R_c	White Powder (EtOH-BuOH)	199-201	$C_{53}H_{90}O_{22}$	3400 (OH) 1620 (C=C)
R_d	White Powder EtOH-AcOEt)	206-9	$C_{48}H_{82}O_{18}$	3400 (OH) 1620 (C=C)
R_e	Colorless needles (50%EtOH)	201-3	$C_{48}H_{82}O_{18}$	3380 (OH) 1620 (C=C)
R_f	White Powder (aceton)	197-8	$C_{42}H_{72}O_{14}$	3380 (OH) 1620 (C=C)
R_{g_1}	Colorless powder	194-6	$C_{42}H_{72}O_{14}$	no OH
R_{g_2}	Colorless powder	187-9	$C_{42}H_{72}O_{13}$	3400 (OH) 1620 (C=C)

Each of these ginsenosides carries a somewhat different sugar molecule, though they all carry monosaccharides. The following table shows the composition of nine ginsenosides of panax ginseng.

Composition of Ginsenosides

Ginsenosides	Prosapogenin (aglycone)	+	Sugar component (mole)
R_{b_0}	Oleanolic acid		glucose (2), glucuronic acid
R_{b_1}	Protopanaxadiol		glucose (4)
R_{b_2}	"		glucose (3), arabinose (1)
R_c	"		glucose (3). arbompse (1)
R_d	"		glucose (3)
R_e	Protopanaxtriol		glucose (2), rhamnose (1)
R_f	"		glucose (2)
R_{g_1}	"		glucose (2)
R_{g_2}	"		glucose (1), rhamnose (1)

The chemical structure of panaxadiol (structure I) was elucidated by Shibata et al., in 1963. In early reports the compounds sapoginol isolated by Kondo et al. in 1915-20, panaxol isolated by Wagner-Jauregg and Roth in 1963,[39] and ginsengenin isolated by Lin,[40] are shown to be identical to panaxadiol.[37]

The structure of protopanaxadiol (structure II) has been confirmed to be an open-chain compound, having a free alcohol group, and an end vinyl group. Drastic acid hydrolysis of protopanaxadiol forms panaxadiol.

The structure of panaxatriol (structure III), similarly, is an acid hydrolyzed product during isolation. The genuine alycone would be protopanaxatriol (structure IV).

Oleanolic acid (structure V) is a pentacyclic, oleanane-type triterpene compound that was initially isolated and identified by Horhammer et al.[41]

The structures of several ginseng saponins, ginsenoside $R_{b\text{-}1}$ (structure VI), ginsenoside $R_{g\text{-}1}$ (structure VII), and

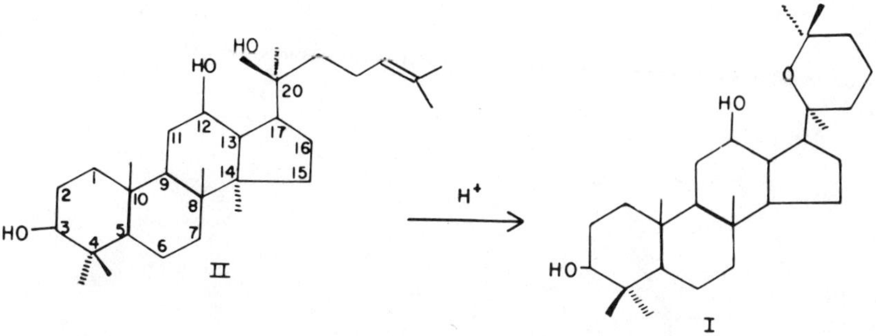
HO
HO
20
12
17
11
13
16
14
15
9
2
1
10
8
HO
3
5
7
4
6
H+
O
HO
HO

II → I

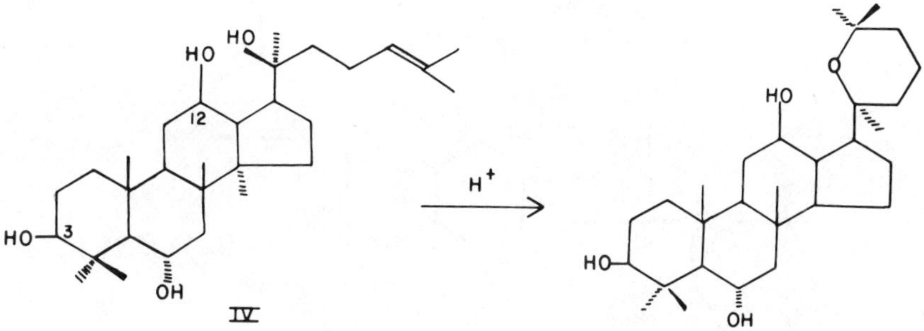
HO
HO
12
HO
3
OH
H+
O
HO
HO
OH

IV → III

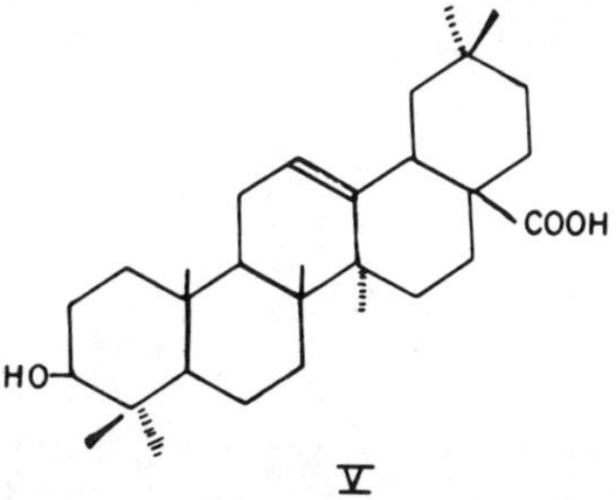
COOH
HO

V

ginsenoside Ro (structure VIII) were eventually established and confirmed. For example, the structure of $R_{g\text{-}1}$ has been established as 6,20-di-O-ß-glucosyl-20-S-protopanaxatriol.

(AGLYCONE)

GINSENOSIDE Rb-I

(SUGAR)   VI

Also confirmed was that panaxoside A, a ginseng saponin isolated by the Soviet chemist, Elyakov *et al.* was identical to ginsenoside R_{g_1},[24]

OTHER COMPONENTS OF GINSENG ROOT

The most important components, other than saponins, from

VII
GINSENOSIDE Rg-1

the extraction of ginseng root are ginseng oil, phytosterol, carbohydrates, acids, nitrogenous substances, vitamins, minerals,
enzymes, and ferments.[17,18,19]

Ginseng Oil and Phytosterol Ginseng oil contains low boiling or volatile, and high boiling or nonvolatile, fractions. The low boiling fraction (boils from 71° to 110°C.) contains panacene and ʟ-elemene. Panacene gives the characteristic fragrance of ginseng. The high boiling fraction (boils from 120° to 150°C.) contains panaxynol.[42,43] Panaxynol, a yellow oil, is a straight-chain, unsaturated alcohol with seventeen carbon atoms.[44,45]

VIII

Ginsenoside R$_0$

(Chikusetsu Saponin V)

β-sitosterol, isolated from the nonvolatile fraction of ginseng oil by Horhammer, is the most common phytosterol in plants.[41] It has been used as a competitive cholesterol inhibitor. Analysis of the phytosterols extracted from Chinese and Korean ginseng revealed that these phytosterols are distinctive for each species.[46] The phytosterol from Chinese ginseng is called stigmasterol,[40] and that from Korean ginseng is called β-sitosterol.[46]

Sugars and Carbohydrates The aqueous extract of ginseng root contains many different types of sugar or saccharide.[47,48,49] The most common single-sugar compounds (monosaccharides) are glucose and fructose. Maltose and sucrose are the most common double-sugars (disaccharides). Multi-sugar compounds such as triasaccharides, tetrasaccharides, and oligosaccharides are also found in ginseng root.

A crude polysaccharide, which was identified as ginseng pectin, was isolated from a boiling-water extract of ginseng root.[50,51,52] Pectin is a high-molecular-weight polysaccharide. It is normally found in plants and fruits. It has been used widely in food preparations such as jellies and jams, as a plasma expander, and medicinally as an antidiarrhea agent.

Organic Acids Many organic acids are present in the alcohol extracts of ginseng roots. The most common organic acids are citric, fumaric, ketoglutaric, oleic, linoleic, linolenic, maleic, malic, pyruvic, succinic, tartaric, and other yet unidentified acids.[53,54] As to ginseng's activity, what role these acids play is not known.

Nonprotein Nitrogenous Substances Nitrogenous substances, about 2%-5% of unknown structure, were detected in the ethereal extract of ginseng root; the nonprotein nitrogenous substance were about 1%-1.5%.[55,56] Although in an early study, it was shown that American ginseng does not contain an alkaloid,[57] a nitrogenous substance called choline has been isolated and identified in the alcoholic extract of ginseng. Choline is an alkaloid in nature; it is found in plants and in animal organs. Choline chloride has been used as lipotropic agent (preventing the excess of accumulation of fat). Choline also gives a marked hypotonic action on blood pressure in rabbits.[58]

Amino Acids and Peptides Korean white ginseng root contains at least fifteen different free amino acids. Some of them are essential and others are nonessential.[59] Essential amino acids are so called because they must be provided by diet, since the body does not manufacture them.[60] The essential amino acids found in ginseng are arginine, histidine, lysine, leucine, threonine, valine, and phenylalanine. Nonessential amino acids, alanine, asparatic acid, glutamic acid, glycine, proline, tyrosine, and serine, are also found in ginseng. Some of these amino acids are found in the stems and leaves, as well as in the root.

Vitamins The ginseng root contains many biologically essential vitamins. So far, vitamin B complex, biotin, niacin, niacinamide, and pantothenic acid have been identified.[61] The presence of vitamin B_{12}, nicotinic acid, and folic acid has also been reported.[62,63] The contents of these vitamins were shown to vary with the age and origin of the ginseng plant.

Minerals and Trace Elements The ginseng root contains many biomedically important mineral and rare element substances. In the water extract of ginseng, elements such as aluminum, manganese, potassium, phosphorus, silicate ions,[64] and sulfur, magnesium, calcium, iron were found.[18,19] The additional minerals and trace elements found were sodium, zinc, copper, molybdenum, and boron.[65]

The trace amount of the rare elements of manganese (Mn), vanadium (V), copper (Cu), cobalt (Co), and arsenic (As) contained in Korean ginseng root were detected by a radioactivation method.[66] These minute amounts of rare elements were found to be extremely important to our health. Ginseng roots cultivated in different areas in Korea contain different amounts of these rare elements.[67]

Trace Element	Korean Ginseng Root Cultivated in			
	Buyo	Kumsan	Kanghwa	Poongki
Manganese	25.9 ppm.*	19.0 ppm.		
Vanadium	0.023 ppm.	0.02 ppm.		
Copper		7.0 ppm.	9.0 ppm.	
Cobalt		0.06 ppm.	0.06 ppm.	
Arsenic		0.44 ppm.		0.25 ppm.

*ppm. = parts per million.

Enzymes Korean fresh ginseng root and dried white root contain diastase, which changes starches into sugars, but the red ginseng root does not.[68] Korean ginseng root also contains other unidentified enzymes and ferments.

GINSENG SAPONINS IN LEAVES AND STEMS

The total crude ginseng saponins vary significantly according to *panax* species, sources of cultivation, and the parts of the plant extracted. Ginseng leaves, stems, and buds contain about 5%-15% of ginseng saponins in comparison to 2%-15% saponins found in roots. Saponin mixtures found in ginseng roots are called ginsenoside R (where R denotes root), while the saponic found in leaves are called ginsenoside F (where F represents folia, meaning leaves).[69,70]

Komatsu and Tomimori isolated fatty acids, nonacosane, and phytosterols from the nonvolatile fraction of the ether extract of ginseng leaves, stems, and flowers. Later, a new natural flavonoid (yellow plant pigment) called panasenoside was isolated and characterized.[71,72]

CONSTITUENTS OF AMERICAN GINSENG

Pioneer studies in Japan showed that American ginseng roots contain many ingredients similar to those found in Korean and Chinese ginseng, but the American root contains slightly more saponin but less proteinous and oily substances.[73,74,75,76] American ginseng also contains inorganic salts (sulfate and phosphate salts of iron, aluminum, and calcium, silicon oxide, and manganese), reducing and nonreducing sugars, phytosterol esters, terpene, panacene, and fatty acids.

Here in the United States, Wong reported his studies on the American ginseng root in 1921. The authentic samples of four- and six-year-old American ginseng roots were crushed and extracted with different solvents. A small amount of ginseng oil, sugar, and saponins were obtained but none contained any alkaloid. By using different organic solvents, quite different amounts of total extractives were obtained. A small amount of enzyme was also detected in the extract, but the nature of the enzyme was not identified. The total extracted ginseng oil was about 0.8 percent.[57] The American ginseng oil was also explored by Torney and Cheng.[78]

In recent years, Professor E. John Staba of the University of Minnesota made extensive studies on American ginseng. He concentrated on the saponins and sapogenins contained in the American ginseng plant. For the first time the saponins of the above-ground parts (stems, leaves, and fruits) of American ginseng were also explored. Jung-yun Kim under the supervision of Professor Staba, earned his Ph. D. from the studies of the phytochemistry of American ginseng in 1974.[79,80] They found that the above-ground parts of the plant contain many of the saponins normally present in the root. The ethereal extract portion contains both beta-sitosterol and stigmasterol. The methanol extract contains predominantly ginseng saponins and saccharides. A total of eleven ginseng saponins, called panaquilins, were isolated and identified. The term *panaquilin* is very similar to *panaquilon*, a name introduced originally by Garriques for the ginseng saponin he isolated from American ginseng root in 1854.[2] These newly isolated American ginseng saponins are panaquilins A, B, C, D, E_1, E_2, E_3, G_1, G_2 (c), and (d). In their studies it was found that the amount of saponins contained in the ginseng plant vary not only with the part of the plant but also with the age of the plant and the season of collection. For example, a six-year-old root contains a different saponin mixture from that found in a two-year-old root. Similarly, the ginseng leaves collected in July contain different saponins from those collected in September. Panaquilins B, C, E_2, E_3, and G_2 are present throughout the plant. Panaquilins D, E_1, and G_1 are present mainly in the root rather than in the above-ground parts; while panaquilins (c), (d), and G_2 are found predominantly in the above-ground parts rather than in the root. The American ginseng leaves contain panaquilins B, C, (d), E_2, E_3, and G_2. After acid hydrolysis of these saponins, sapogenins (aglycones) were obtained.

Dr. Staba carefully compared the properties of panaquilins with those of ginsenosides (isolated by Shibata *et al.*) and panaxosides (isolated by Elyakov *et al.*) and found that the American ginseng root has a different composition of ginseng saponins. The following table gives the comparison of these ginseng saponins.

Similarities of Panaquilins, Ginsenosides, and Panaxosides
Isolated from American and Korean Ginseng Roots

Plant Species:	American Ginseng *(Panax quinquefolium)*		Panax ginseng
Panaquilin	*Ginsenoside* (Japanese terminology)		*Panaxoside* (Russian terminology)
—	R_o		—
—	R_a		F
B	R_{b-1}	R_{b-2}	E
C	R_c		D
D	R_d		—
E_1	-		—
E_2	R_d		C
E_3	R_e		B
—	R_f		—
G_1	R_{g-1}		A
G_2	R_{g-2}		—
—	R_{g-3}		—
—	R_{h-1}		—
—	R_{h-2}		—

Although *P. ginseng* and American ginseng contain similar ginseng saponins, panaquilins E_1 and G_2 (in American ginseng) are absent in the root of *P. Ginseng*; while ginsenosides R_a and R_f are not present in the root of American ginseng. The American ginseng root contains about 17.3% panaxadiol, 0.44% panaxatriol, and about 0.28% oleanolic acid. The approximate ratio of panaxadiol to panaxatriol of American ginseng root is about 39 to 1 by column chromatography, or 40 to 1 by preparative chromatography. On the other hand, the ratio of sapogenin panaxadiol to panaxatriol for *P. ginseng* is about equal. Accordingly, the American ginseng contains much more panaxadiol than *P. ginseng* root.[79,80] This could be the reason why the Chinese have always said that American ginseng is different in medicinal properties from *Panax ginseng*, or Chinese ginseng.

CONSTITUENTS OF JAPANESE GINSENG

Japanese ginseng (*Panax japonicum* C. A. Meyer) is also called *chikusetzu ninjim* in Japanese. It has been the most widely used ginseng substitute in Japan, chiefly for stomachic, expectorant, and antipyretic action.

Inuoue[4] seemed to be the first who reported finding and testing pharmacologically a saponin isolated from Japanese ginseng in 1902. Later Murayama *et al.*,[81,82] Aoyama,[83] and Kotake *et al.*,[84] also investigated the crude ginseng saponin. Kitasota *et al.*[85] and Kuwata and Matsukawa[86] isolated oleanolic acid from Japanese ginseng. In 1962, Shibata *et al.* reported that in addition to oleanolic acid, arabinose, glucose, and glucuronic acid, a small amount of panaxadiol was also preent in saponin mixture isolated from Japanese ginseng.[28]

Professors Kondo *et al.* isolated three saponins; *chikusetsu* saponins III, IV, and V in crystalline forms and also confirmed the structures of these saponins.[87] *Chikusetsu* saponin III is composed of protopanaxadiol or 20-epi-protopanaxadiol, and glucoses (2 moles), and xylose. This particular saponin is a homologous saponin of ginsenoside found in *Panax ginseng*. *Chikusetsu* saponin IV is composed of oleanolic acid bound with glucose, arabinose and glucuronic acid. *Chikusetsu* saponin V is also an oleanolic acid bound with glucoses (2 moles) and glucuronic acid. This particular saponin is found to be identical with ginsenoside R_o of ginseng saponin.

The structure of *chikusetsu* saponin IV is shown to be identical to a tonic saponin of araloside A, which was isolated from *Aralia manschuria*, Araliaceae, by Kochetkov *et al.*[88]

CONSTITUENTS OF HIMALAYAN GINSENG

Eight saponins, namely, saponins A, B, C, D, E, F, G, and H, have been successfully isolated, and among them saponin A and saponin D have been identified.[89]

Hydrolysis of saponin A, a white powder, in dilute HCl gives oleanolic acid, glucose, and glucuronic acid. From chemical and physical data, it has been confirmed that saponin A is identical to *chikusetsu* saponin V, the main saponin of *P. japonicum* C. A. Meyer.

Saponin D, also, is a white powder, and the IR spectra showed the presence of hydroxyl and olefinic bonds. The acid hydrolysis of saponin D with HCl-dioxane-water gave panaxadiol and glucose, which were identified by TLC, paper partition chromatography, and gas liquid chromatography. It consists of 20-protopanaxadiol and four moles of glucose. Saponin D has been confirmed to be identical to ginsenoside R_{b-1}, the chief saponin present in ginseng root.

The hydrolyzed products of saponins showed some differences among the different ginseng species. Japanese and Himalayan ginseng roots contain mainly oleanane-type triterpenes, while ginseng and American ginseng roots contain more dammarane-type triterpenes glycosides.[76]

It is very interesting to note that the leaves of many *Panax* species such as Chinese ginseng, Japanese ginseng, Himalayan ginseng, as well as American ginseng, contain a cetain amount of many of the saponins present in the roots.[69,79] The Chinese ginseng leaves contain more panaxadiol and panaxatriol but little oleanolic acid. On the other hand, the leaves of Japanese ginseng contain more panaxatriol and oleanolic acid but little panaxadiol, while Himalayan ginseng leaves contain more panaxadiol.[76]

CONSTITUENTS OF SIBERIAN GINSENG

Siberian ginseng (*Eleutherococcus senticosus* of Araliaceae) contains many biologically active saponin glycosides. At least six glycosides, called *eleutherosides*, have been isolated from the root of Siberian ginseng. Eleutherosides A, B, C, D, E, and F are known and have been tested in animals.[90,91]

Eleutheroside A has been identified as daucosterin, Eleutherosides B, D, and E are structurally close, and they all are syringarosinol. Eleutheroside C is a nonglycoside, while Eleutherosides A, B, D, and E contain aglycones of varied structures. Eleutheroside F is of unknown structure.[92]

10

HOW GINSENG WORKS

Ginseng's value as a universal tonic, which promotes and maintains good health, particularly for those who are physically and mentally troubled, aged men and women, has long been recognized in the Orient, and is slowly gaining recognition in the Western world. For quite a long time Chinese medical practice has claimed that ginseng has the power to restore vigor, maintain health, and erase the debilities of old age. Numerous scientific experiments in laboratories and clinical trials in humans have helped to establish that ginseng preparations are indeed capable of stimulating the functions and regulating the malfunctions of the organs, the central nervous system, the cardiovascular system, the endocrine glands, and the metabolism.[1] In addition, ginseng is unique in medicinal properties in that it remarkably increases an organism's resistance to harmful stresses arising from various origins, thus maintaining the normal functions of the organism.[2]

For thousands of years the Chinese as well as other Orientals used ginseng, primarily, for *tonic* purposes. Chinese doctors believe that most ailments are due to the debility of the body or the lost of balance or harmony of the organism. Accordingly, for mental and physical debility ginseng is the best remedy. On the other hand, Soviet scientists have confirmed that ginseng is a harmless *adaptogen*. The real truth about ginseng, the evidence on "how ginseng works", and "what ginseng can do for you" are discussed in the following chapters.

157

ADAPTOGENIC POWER OF GINSENG

The distinguished pharmacologist Dr. I. I. Brekhman and his associates of the Institute of Biologically Active Substances, Siberian Branch of the Academy of Sciences of the USSR, Vladivostok, have been conducting systemic biological research on Oriental herb drugs, particularly ginseng and Siberian ginseng, for more than twenty-five years. Evidence from laboratory and clinical investigations indicates that the basic effect of ginseng's activity is its capacity to increase the nonspecific resistance of the organism toward various stresses.[3,4,5] This characteristic medical claim is called *adaptogenic activity*. The concept of adaptogenic activity represents a recent innovation in Western medicine, a new milestone in modern therapeutics.

Adaptogen According to Drs. Brekhman and Dardymov, *Panax ginseng* and several other species of the Araliaceae family provide the medical properties of adaptogens.[4,5] The word *adaptogen* means "a substance causing a state of nonspecifically increased resistance of the organism to stresses of various origin." Ginseng is one of the most useful adapteogens.[5] The concept of "a state of nonspecifically increased resistance (SNIR)" of the organism was originally developed by N. V. Lazarev, who found that 2-benzyl-benzimidazol (bendazol) was effective for the treatment of damage to various regions of the nervous system, and for increasing nonspecific resistance of the organism to adverse stresses.[6] As a matter of fact, the recent discovery of the adaptogenic activity of bendazol and its analogous drugs was preceeded long ago in well-established Oriental herb medicine.

Requirements To Be an Adaptogen What type of medicinal agents have the virtue of adaptogens? The requirements for a remedy to be an adaptogen, according to Dr. Brekhman, are that it should be: (1) innocuous or safe; (2) have antistress activities; and (3) possess normalizing and protective effects. According to published research reports, ginseng and Siberian ginseng (Eleuthero) meet all the fundamental requirements necessary to be classified as adaptogens. One of the most important indices of a drug's adaptogenic action is its capacity to increase a human's physical resistance toward adverse stresses and maintain the body in homeostasis.[5] Thus, ginseng overcomes diseases by a mechanism of building the general vitality and resistance, and by strengthening the normal functions of the organism. Dr. Brekhman proclaimed that ginseng, without any doubt, is an "adaptogen," if not a "panacea."[5]

THE HARMLESS MANROOT

When we use a drug, we want to know its purity, side effects, and its relative toxicity and safety. The laboratory LD_{50} index, or fifty percent animal lethal (death) dosage, is the method most frequently used in pharmacology and toxicology to indicate the toxicity of the drug.

After repeated tests, it has been proved that ginseng root, its extracts, and its chemically purified constituents (ginseng saponins) are harmless. The well-known ginseng pharmacologists Drs. Brekhman,[5] Yonekawa,[7] Kitagawa and Iwaki,[8] Hong,[9] and Kaku, et al.[10] have repeatedly stressed the fact that ginseng has a very low toxicity in comparison with a majority of commonly used *official* remedies. Yonekawa[7] found that the lethal dose of ginseng saponin, ginsenin, was 2-3 g/kg. in mice, while Kitagawa and Iwaki[8] found that the LD_{50} of ginseng ethereal extract in mice was 5 g/kg. Brekhman[5] reported that the LD_{50} of *Panax ginseng* root was 10-30 g/kg., while the LD_{50} for the isolated pure ginseng saponins, panaxosides, given orally were 1.4 g/kg. in mice. The oral toxicity of ginseng root is about ten to twenty times less than that of its pure saponins. Even for the pure ginseng saponins, the LD_{50} of gensenoside R_{g-1} is 1.25 g/kg, given intraperitoneally to mice.[10] The toxicity of ginseng saponin is similar or lower than those of most commonly used *official* drugs. For example, the oral LD_{50} value (in rats) of aspirin is 1.75 g/kg.; caffeine, 0.2 g/kg.: and sulfaquanidine (an intestinal antibacterial agent), 1.0 g/kg. Thus, ginseng is an *innocuous* and perhaps even a safer remedy in comparison with those officially accepted as "drugs."

STRESS AND ANTISTRESS ACTIVITY OF GINSENG

What Is Stress? Stress, in a broad sense, is mental or physical strain, pressure, tension, or unhappiness. Frustration and suffering are also stressful conditions. Adverse stresses can be man-made or due to the environment. The most common chemical and physical sources of stress are drugs, chemicals, fumes, polluted water and air, high or low pressures, extreme temperatures, and radiation. Biological causes of stress may be bacteria, toxins, foreign sera, viruses, and tumor tissue. In addition to these physical environmental and biological stresses, there are also mental stresses of a socioeconomic nature.

Stress can make you miserable or ill. In extreme cases, it can kill you. But how do you respond to stress? For a long time, doctors have told us to avoid stress, but Dr. Hans Selye, considered the world's leading authority on stress, says that the key to handling stress is to work at something at which you can win. You can overcome the effects of stress by following a code of behavior based on natural laws.[11]

Stress-Related Diseases Evidence is growing that stress can be one of the components of any disease. The presence of stressful environmental conditions is one of the major factors that contribute to an individual's susceptibility to disease, as pointed out by Dr. Robert Ader, Professor of Psychiatry and Psychology at the University of Rochester School of Medicine and Dentistry.[12]

"Every illness from the common cold to cancer, has a psychologic component," said Dr. Samuel Silverman, Associate Clinical Professor of Psychiatry at Harvard Medical School. Some physicians, including Dr. Silverman, still think that the seven well-defined diseases [peptic ulcer, hypertension, hyperthyroidism, rhumatoid arthritis, ulcerative colitis, neurodermatitis and asthma], are *psychosomatic* diseases, that is, the physical disorder is caused by the emotional state of the patient.[12]

How Your Body Handles Stress Laboratory studies on animals have shown that the adrenal gland in particular is the prime reactor to stress. For example, when rats are exposed to various types of stress such as environmental temperature change, pressure change, injecting foreign protein or toxic material, all the rats had their adrenals enlarged, while the lymph nodes, thymus, spleen, gastric and duodenal tract had shrunk. The initial response of the body to any kind of stress is alarm, followed by the stage of resistance.

Professor Selye, the world-famous endocrinologist and director of the American Academy of Stress Disorders, published his original concept of reactions toward stress, the "nonspecific biological stress syndrome" describing the pituitary-adrenal axis that releases powerful corticosteroids in the body's precautionary girding for "fight or flight" when responding to danger or startle.[12]

Typical Stress Examples Stress, such as meeting the annual income tax return deadline of April 15, may lead to serious physiological changes, which may even result in cardiovascular disorders. Drs. Meyer Friedman and Ray Roseman of Mount Zion Hospital and Medical Center followed the blood changes of eighteen tax accountants between January and June. As a rule, the accountants increased their workload to seventy-hour weeks against the April target date, then slacked off to leisurely thirty-hour weeks. In the course of this experiment, the group's serum cholesterol averaged 206 mg% to 217 mg% during the off-season winter months of work, rose sharply in March, and peaked at a mean 323 mg% by mid-April. Then by the first week in June, it declined to 206 mg%. Blood clotting times kept pace, from 8.1 minutes in February, dropping to a tense, taut 5 minutes on April 15, and by June increased again to 8.8 minutes. This economical stress on the accountants caused high blood cholesterol, one of the effects of stress in persons prone to cardiovascular disorders.[13]

Both Drs. Sidney Cobb of Brown University and Robert Rose of Boston University School of Medicine agree that because of the round-the-clock and day-in and day-out stress of split-second decisions and actions, air-traffic controllers have a higher-than-average incidence of hypertension, peptic ulcers, and diabetes.[14] Hypertension has long been thought to be a psychosomatic disease — the disease caused by stress. Elevated blood pressure has been specifically associated with emergency situations, with prolonged combat duty, and with job termination.[14]

How would unemployment affect one's health? In 1975, the unemployment rate was headed for ten percent nationwide, but in an economic disaster area such as Detroit, the automobile city, fifteen to twenty percent of the work force was idle. Dr. Gordon Deshler, medical director of Detroit's Metropolitan Health plan, said: "The truth of the matter is that Detroit is probably one of the most stressful areas in the whole world. We have large numbers of people who require continuing support with medication for pain, anxiety, for stress, and so forth. It really is pretty much a way of life."[12]

Antistress Effect of Ginseng Quite a number of interesting laboratory investigations dealing with the protective or antistress effect of ginseng have been reported in medical literature. It is of great interest and importance that some properties of ginseng are demonstrable only in stressed, injured, and impaired animals. In other words, normal animals or animals kept at normal conditions usually show little or no physiological change after being fed ginseng. This is because animals usually retain their homeostasis. Therefore, in order to evaluate the true anti-stress effect of ginseng, various types of experiments were designed using animals under severe stress or animals with previously induced stresses of a physical, chemical, or biological nature.

Physical stresses, such as extremely cold and hot temperatures, have been used to evaluate how the animals react, and what role ginseng plays in the reaction to stress. Quantitative measurements of the vitamin C (ascorbic acid) content in the adrenal gland of the test animals and their body temperature have been used as indicators to evaluate stress. This is because under extreme temperatures, either cold or hot, the adrenal vitamin C of the animals usually falls to a very low level.

It seems that the earliest laboratory studies on temperature stress started some twenty years ago. In 1958, two Chinese physiologists, Sung and Chi of the Chinese Academy of Medical Sciences, Peking, announced their fundamental research discovery on the protective effect of ginseng against temperature stresses.[15] In their study, white male rats were divided into two groups: one group ate a regular diet, while the other group ate the same diet supplemented with 5% ginseng powder. After three weeks, some of the rats from both groups were put into a 78-90°C chamber for five to six minutes or put into a chamber of -2°C. for one hour before being returned to room temperature. In another experiment, each rat received 2.4 ml of fifty percent ginseng extract one hour before the temperature stress, while rats fed with water served as controls. After temperature stress, all of the rats were killed and the vitamin C content of their adrenal glands was determined. It was found that the vitamin C (ascorbic acid) content of the adrenal glands of rats subjected to either hot or cold temperature stress was significantly depleted. However, the depletion of the adrenal vitamin C was less in rats treated with ginseng powder in their diet or with ginseng extract one hour before the stress. Also, the rats in the control group subjected to high temperature stress either appeared unable to move or showed chronic convulsion, and did not regain their normality until twenty to sixty minutes after their removal from the hot chamber. On the other hand, most of the rats fed with ginseng appeared to be normal immediately after their removal from the hot chamber and none of them showed convulsion. Their work clearly indicated that ginseng was capable of increasing the nonspecific resistance of the organism to temperature stress. The authors suggested that the administration of ginseng extract may interfere with the nervous control of the pituitary gland or that ginseng has adrenocorticotropic hormon (ACTH)-like action.[15,16]

Similar antistress effects observed with ginseng could in some cases also be obtained with cortisol or cortisone. Thus, the question has been raised whether the antistress effects of ginseng are actually mediated through the adrenal cortex or through the brain pituitary-adrenal cortex system. Studies in the area of endocrinology are very difficult. Many times, Dr. I. I. Brekhman has said that the intravenous injection of ginseng extract to a dying cat, after it has lost its breath and heart beat, can often revive it. Chang and Kao injected a ginseng extract to dogs dying as a result of bleeding or suffocation, and brought the dogs to life. All these indicate that the action of ginseng is definitely related to the adrenal system or the pituitary gland of the brain or both.[17]

In 1964, the effect of ginseng against temperature stress was investigated by Drs. Tsung, Chen, and Tang of Kirin Medical Institute.[18] In their experiments, instead of measuring the adrenal vitamin C level, they explored the possible mechanism of the organism's antistress activity by observing how the animal survived. Ninety-two male white mice, were treated by intraperitoneal injection of a fifty percent aqueous extract of ginseng, 10 ml/kg, to each mouse; while those injected with same amount of physiological saline were served as controls. In each experiment, six mice (three experimental and three control) were put into a 45-47°C. chamber thirty minutes after the injection or into a -2°C. chamber twenty minutes after the injection. The mice were allowed to remain in the chamber until half of the mice were dead. The results showed that out of twenty-one mice in each group, fourteen mice in the control group and seven in the experimental group were dead under heat stress while among the twenty-five mice in each group kept in the cold chamber, eighteen in the control group and six in the experimental group were dead. In a second series of experiments, the adrenals of the mice were taken out and by a similar procedure, they were put in the cold and hot temperature chambers. The results showed that out of seventeen mice in each group, seven in the control group and ten in the experimental group were dead in the hot chamber, while out of twenty mice in each group ten in the control group and nine in the experimental group were dead under cold stress. Their experiments clearly confirmed that ginseng strikingly raised the animals' ability to tolerate temperature stress, and elongated their survival under stress. However, this antistress activity was abolished after the removal of the adrenals. The authors then suggested that the mechanism of the antistress activity of the organism induced after the injection of ginseng might be associated with the hypophysis (pituitory gland)-adrenal system.[18]

Research on the antistress activity of ginseng was also pursued in Bulgaria. In 1963, Petkov and Staneva-Stoicheva of Post-graduate Medical Institute, Sofia, reported their work on the effect of ginseng on the adrenal cortex.[19] In their experiments, white rats were fed with twenty percent alcoholic extract of ginseng by means of a stomach tube at daily dose of 2 ml/kg, for seventeen days, while a second group of rats, fed with the same volume of water, served as controls. In one series of their experiments, they found that the eosinophil count in the peripheral blood of the experimental rats was twenty-six percent lower than at the beginning of the experiment. The control animals had only a slight reduction in the number of eosinophil cells. The average weight of the adrenals of the experimental rats was increased by about thirteen percent over that of the controls. Also there was a slight decrease in the vitamin C content of the adrenal cortex but the corticosteroid content in the urine was found to be sixty percent higher in the experimental animals than in the controls. Another series of experiments were performed under hot stress by immersing one hind leg of the rat in hot water (70^{0}C) for one minute. Ater this stress, the eosinophil count of the control animals had a forty-one percent rise after two hours and a forty-five percent rise after four hours of the stress, while the rats under ginseng treatment, after the same intervals, showed a twelve percent and a nine percent fall of the eosinophil count. During the subsequent days three rats in the control group died while all the rats in the experimental group survived. In a third series of experiments, all of the rats had one of their adrenal glands removed (adrenalectomy). After this unilateral adrenalectomy, the remaining adrenal gland of the ginseng-treated rats, in each case, weighed much more than the adrenal gland that had been removed at the beginning of the experiment. The corresponding increase in weight of the adrenal gland of the rats in the control group was insignificant. Accordingly, the hypertrophy effect (enlargement) of the adrenal gland of the experimental rats indicates the pharmacological action of ginseng. All these results, according to Dr. Petkov, confirmed that ginseng extract had a stimulating effct on the adrenal cortex and this effect may be of neurogenic origin. Ginseng increased the reactivity of the cerebro-cortical cells thus facilitating the adaptation of adrenal cortical function to the needs of the organism under stress. The antiinflammatory and antiexudative effects of ginseng, as had been reported by others, may be also due to the stimulating effect of ginseng on glycocorticoid hormone production.[19]

After the studies of Sung and Chi, Tsung and associates, and Petkov, Wang of the Chinese Medicine Research Institute in Kirin further reported that a twenty percent alcoholic extract of ginseng leaves and stems had a stimulating effect on the activities of the pituitary-adrenal cortex system. From different pharmacological experiments, Wang confirmed that the activity of ginseng was not directly on the adrenal cortex *per se* but rather on the cerebral level, that is, the pituitary gland of the brain.[20]

In recent years, studies on the antistress effect of ginseng were performed in much greater detail by many investigators in South Korea. For example, in 1964, B. I. Kim reported that an alcoholic extract of ginseng, as does hydrocortisone, prolonged the survival time of the adrenalectomized mice when exposed to cold.[21] In 1965, C. Kim reported that the total serum protein, hemoglobin, and the red blood cells of mice were markedly decreased when exposed to a cold environment. However, the ginseng-treated mice, on the other hand, showed an increase in the serum hemoglobin and the red blood cell counts.[22] In 1965, G. C. Kim reported the influence of ginseng on the rectal temperature of mice in a cold environment in comparison with cortisone and chloropromazine.[23] In his experiments, 1,680 mice were divided into four groups: a normal group without restraint (movement of all four legs were uninhibited), a normal group with restraint, adrenalectomized mice without restraint, and adrenalectomized mice with restraint. These mice were exposed to a cold temperature of $0°C$ (fifty minutes per day) for one, five, and ten days. The adrenalectomy (both sides) was performed three days before the cold stress. It was found that the mice treated with ginseng (an alcoholic exract at a daily dose of 20 mg/kg) and treated with cortisone (at a dose of 10 mg/kg/day) repressed the drop of rectal temperature of all groups and the supression effect was more apparent with the mice in the restraint groups. Both ginseng and cortisone exerted a greater effect upon the normal mice than the adrenalectomized mice in preventing the rectal temperature drop. It is surprising, however, after the administration of chloropromazine (a dose level of 9.5 mg/kg/day), that both the normal and adrenalectomized mice with restraint showed a further drop in the rectal temperature.[23]

Similar studies on the influence of ginseng upon the rectal temperature of rats exposed to cold was also reported by Yoon and Kim in 1971. Two hundred adult male albino rats were divided into ginseng and saline groups. For eight or fifteen consecutive days, the rats received 5 ml/kg of either a ginseng extract or a physiological saline. The significant findings from their studies were: without exposure to cold environment, there was no significant difference in rectal temperature between the ginseng and the saline groups, regardless of whether the rats were intact (without any surgery), hypophysectomized, adrenalectomized, thyroidectomized, or thyroid-adrenalectomized; the rectal temperature of the ginseng-treated rats after the different types of surgery as mentioned above dropped little in comparison with those in the saline group; also ginseng facilitated the earlier recovery from abnormal to normal rectal temperature than saline in the rats under cold stress.[24]

Hu and associates reported their series of studies on the effect of ginseng against temperature stresses. Their findings were essentially similar to those reported by others indicating that ginseng exerted little or no influence upon the adrenal vitamin C content of animals under normal temperature conditions. However, the administration of ginseng did accelerate the recovery from, and helped the maintenance of, the body temperature under cold or heat stress conditions. [25,26,27,28,29]

Only recently W. B. Kim, H. R. Kim and H. Y. Chung found that after the administration of ACTH, the adrenal vitamin C content decreased significantly as it does with temperature stress. However, animals, both mature and immature, under the influence of ginseng showed a protective effect and mitigated the fall in the adrenal vitamin C content.[30,31]

Ever since the announcement of ginseng's adaptogenic power by Brekhman, scientists all over the world tried to prove and also disprove its marvelous action. Amirov and Abdulova reported that the increase in the resistance of the body to toxic substances can be achieved not only by gradual adaptation to toxic substances but also by the administration of ginseng. As an adaptogen, ginseng has polytropic action. It improves the resistance of the body toward stresses by any mechanism that may act upon the endocrine system, metabolic processes, and may be joined together with neurohumoral mechanisms, thus stimulating the amazing defensive or adaptive activities of the body.[32]

The tendency to get sick and also the ill effects of exposure to toxic chemicals such as morphine, cocaine, strychnine, and curare poisons were much less in ginseng-fed animals than in control animals.[33,34,35] Animals under ginseng treatment also showed relatively longer survival time during periods of starvation,[36] or when exposed to low pressure and extremely cold temperature after adrenal gland removal.[37] The tolerance of ginseng-treated mice to the stress of increased gravitational force was greater than that of the control group,[38,39] another incident showing the antistress effect of ginseng.

NORMALIZING EFFECT OF GINSENG

The third and most important attribute of an adaptogen is its normalizing effect upon wounds and fast recovery from various illnesses. In experimental investigations with animals, it has been established that ginseng is effective against chemically (alloxan)-induced diabetes, radiation sickness, experimental emotional disorders, mental strain and nervous exhaustion, hypotension, and certain forms of hypertension and cancer.[5] This broad-spectrum antistress effect of ginseng is due to its normalizing effect. The so-called normalizing effect of ginseng or of any other adaptogenic drug is a new dimension in medicine and a novel approach in therapeutics. The following are a few examples to illustrate the marvelous normalizing effect of ginseng.

Liver damage caued by carbon tetrachloride or irradiation was prevented by the administration of ginseng extract to animals.[40] Ginseng also prevented the development of fever induced by intravenous injection of typhoid and a paratyphoid vaccine in rabbits. When mice were injected with trypanosomes (a genus of flagellate protozoan), it was found that the life span of the ginseng-treated animals was significantly prolonged compared to that of the controls.[40] Rabbits innoculated with *Shigella paradysenteriae* W. and given ginseng extract suffered only from a drastically increased number of leukocytes (white blood cells) in the blood, whereas the control animals developed diseased white blood cells (leukopenia).[41]

Ginseng has certain antiinflammatory activities. It appears to be capable of lessening the swelling at the ankle joints due to the injection of egg-white or dextran.[42] A noticeable antiinflammatory effect was obtained in rabbits having an inflammation of the ear-shell caused by freezing.

In general, laboratory experimental work revealed that in animals exposed to pathological environmental conditions, the ginseng-fed animals showed quick adjustment with respect to the adverse conditions. This is the typical normalizing of the organism under the influence of ginseng. In addition to the medical defensive power, the wonder root is further capable of aiding in recovery from damage such as abnormal enlargment (hypertrophy) and contraction (atrophy) of the adrenal and thyroid glands caused by toxic chemicals; reducing the blood sugar level in animals having very high blood sugar; or increasing the blood sugar level in animals having very low blood sugar. The normalization effect was also attained in red blood cell diseases as well as white blood cell diseases.[43,44]

After learning all the facts about ginseng's mysterious adaptogenic power, we know no chemical drug today that is comparable to ginseng. No wonder the manroot deserves the title of "panacea," or "elixir of life," and has been scientifically called "adaptogen." In my opinion, to maintain homeostasis and good health we all need this mysterious adaptogen against all known and unknown harmful stresses and distresses.

11

WHAT GINSENG CAN DO FOR YOU

A SAFE TONIC AND THE ANTIFATIGUE EFFECT OF GINSENG

Fatigue Fatigue is the common symptom of weariness that occurs after sustained or intensive physical or mental strain. Fatigue causes irritability, decreased ability to concentrate, a tendency to be upset by trivialities, and impairment of the ability to rationalize. Most often, psychiatric fatigue, such as combat fatigue during a period of war, is a very common sympton of distress, uneasiness, or emotional disorders. Common symptoms associated with these disorders are headache, chest pain, very rapid beating of the heart, along with a difficulty in breathing. Certain illnesses such as anemia, chronic infection, malnutrition, metabolic disease, and endocrine gland disorders, may cause chronic fatigue.

Tonic Effect of Ginseng Repeated laboratory tests have shown that the active principles of ginseng root indeed are able to prevent fatigue and to increase the physical performance of animals, including man. "The increase in strength and efficiency after a single dose is called *stimulant action*, while the improved vitality after prolonged administration of ginseng is called *tonic effect,* according to Dr. Brekhman.[1]

The stimulant effect of ginseng was first tested in humans by the Chinese two thousand years ago. The test consisted of a person with a piece of ginseng root in his mouth walking for 5 *li* while another walked with his mouth empty, and if the person with ginseng in his mouth did not feel tired or out of breath, the root in his mouth was genuine ginseng (the tonic effect). The other person must be out of breath. This two-man-walk test was the first trial in history to identify if the ginseng was genuine or an adulterant.

The first modern method of detecting the *tonic* and *antifatigue* effect of ginseng in animals was a swimming test using white mice of similar weight.[2,3,4,5] In order to make the results more obvious and the testing period of swimming shorter, a 1 g. weight was put on the tails of the mice. Results from hundreds of tests showed that the average swimming time after oral administration or injection of 0.15 ml. of ginseng extract, was increased to about sixty to one hundred percent over controls.[1,3,5]

The antifatigue effect of ginseng is more pronounced if ginseng has been taken continuously for a longer time. Again, by using the swimming test with mice, Soviet scientists conducted experiments that continued for two months, during which time the mice had to swim once every five days. For the first ten days on which they swam, no ginseng preparation was given. From the eleventh day to the fortieth day, half of the mice received injections in an amount of 0.1 ml. per mouse (20 g. of body weight) of a ten percent aqueous liquid extract once every other day. Mice in control received two percent alcohol solution. The swimming was started twenty minutes after the injection. At the end of the two-month test, the average swimming time of the mice in control was about 47-61 min., while those under the influence of ginseng was about 96-117 min., which is about an eighty percent improvement. It was further noted that in the twenty-mouse groups, eight in the control group and only four in the ginseng-treated group were dead as a result of complete physical exhaustion.[6]

A second method is to measure the increased duration of running on a endless rope.[7] The device consists of four closed, vertical boxes $7 \times 7 \times 25$ cm. Through the center of each box, a descending rope is passed. The rope is put into motion by an electric motor at a velocity of about 6 m./min. The floors of the boxes are electrified to about twenty-five volts. The time to complete fatigue is that time when the mice can no longer run, but remain on the floor despite the current being on. In this particular test, the mice under the influence of ginseng gave a significantly better performance than the control.

In order to test the potency of the ginseng preparations, the amount of the preparation that increases the work duration by about thirty three percent is called one "Stimulant Unit of Action" denoted as SUA_{33}.[6] This particular pharmacological testing method of ginseng preparations was developed by Dr. I. I. Brekhman at Vladivostok. It was shown that the active principles, ginseng saponin glycosides isolated by Soviet chemists from the Chinese ginseng root, gave much more pronounced stimulant action than the crude extract. This ws proved by the swimming and rope-running tests.[8] One stimulant unit of action (SUA_{33}) equals 0.101 ml./20 g. of body weight of fifteen percent solution of ginseng extract, or 0.151 mg. of ginseng saponin glycoside, panaxoside C, powder. A number of ginseng saponins and aglycones (obtained after acid hydrolysis of saponins) isolated from the ginseng root are about 100 to 1,000 times more potent than the crude extract. Among the five ginseng saponins isolated by the Soviet chemists, panaxosides A and C (panaxatriol group) are more potent than panaxosides D, E, and F (panaxadiol group). Also, panaxoside C, with four sugar molecules, is twice as potent as panaxoside A, which has only three sugar molecules. The aglycone, panaxatriol, possesses a relatively higher activity than panaxadiol. Of the panaxadiols, panaxoside D is the most potent. Panaxoside E and panaxoside F are a pentoxide and a hexoside, respectively, and are less active than panaxoside D. The potencies of panaxosides are about 700-6,600 SUA_{33}, while the potencies of the aglycones are about 2,000 to 5,000 SUA_{33} in comparison with ginseng extracts which are only 50 to 70 SUA_{33}.[3] Furthermore, the activities of ginseng extracts from natural ginseng were virtually the same as those cultivated ginseng roots.

The Japanese workers, without delay, repeated the swimming tests of mice conducted initially by the Soviet investigators; however, a slightly different approach was adopted. In the tests, four different types of ginseng extracts were used, i.e., ether extract, alcohol extract, water total extract (without previously extracting with organic solvents), and water extract (after extraction with ether). Five mice in a group were to swim at 32⁰C. until exhaustion, and the swimming performance of each mouse was recorded. As is shown in the following table, with the mice in the control groups the duration of swimming was from 34 (shortest) to 194 (longest) seconds, while with the mice after treatment with ginseng extract, the swimming performance was significantly increased. It was especially noted that the mice treated with alcohol extract, ether extract, and water extract respectively showed the swimming duration, in each case, to be improved by from sixty to two hundred percent in comparison to both the shortest and the longest swimming records of the controls. Particularly noteworthy was the comparison between the performance observed one hour after treatment with ginseng extract to that conducted three days after the oral treatment with ginseng extract. Thus one hour after treatment with ginseng the mice's performances were much better than the controls.[5]

The antifatigue effect of ginseng was also tested using special commercially available ginseng preparations* of GI Phar-

Swimming Performance in Mice with and without Ginseng Extract Treatment*

		Ether Extract	Alcohol Extract	Total Water Extract	Control group I	Control group II	Control group III
Dose in mg/kg.		200	100	100			
	Test A	55-123	52-164	80-198	34-96	40-96	46-194
Duration of Swimming (in Seconds							
	Test B	74-280	131-577	104-242	40-116	41-101	52-180

*The swimming tests were performed at 32⁰C., 5 mice in a group. The durations of swimming (from the shortest to the longest) were recorded, and are shown in the Table. A represents the swimming tests conducted three days after oral administration of the ginseng extract; B represents the swimming tests conducted one hour after administration of the ginseng extract.

*Pharmaton, Ltd. Lugano, Switzerland.

maton and Geriatric Pharmaton. The swimming time of rats after administration of these preparations was significantly prolonged over controls. Geriatric Pharmaton gave a much more pronounced effect than the GI Pharmaton preparation.[9]

The most recent mice swimming studies were performed by Dr. K. H. Rueckert of Pharmaton, Ltd., Lugano, Switzerland.[10] In his first experiment, 450 mice were used. These mice, both male and female of similar body weight of about twenty grams, were divided into nine groups of fifty mice each. The swimming performance of these mice was measured after the mice had been treated with Pharmaton's ginseng extract in the diet. Two dose levels of the ginseng extract were used, i.e., 3 mg/kg/day or 0.06 mg/20 g. (mouse body weight), and 30 mg/kg/day or 0.6 mg/20 g. Each of these dose levels was administered continuously to groups of mice for periods of fourteen, twenty-one, and twenty-eight days. At each time interval, the swimming performance of the ginseng-treated mice was tested and compared with that of the untreated control group. In the swimming test, the mice were placed in a water bath at 18°C and allowed to swim until complete exhaustion. The swimming time of each mouse was recorded. After the first swim, the mice were allowed to dry out in a warm air stream. Each mouse was then retested after a rest-drying period of one hour. When the swimming tests were completed, the average or mean swimming time in each of the two tests of the two dose groups was computed. The results showed that the mice treated with 0.06 mg/day dose for fourteen days improved little, while the mice treated with 0.6 mg/day had better swimming performance than the control group. The improvement was about twelve to twenty percent. After twenty one days of tretment with ginseng extract, the swimming performance of 0.6 mg/day group was about twenty seven percent better at the first test and about twenty percent better at the second test than the control group. After twenty-eight days of ginseng extract treatment, the swimming performance was significantly improved by about forty-eight percent at the first test, and about thirty eight percent at the second test over the control group; the mice treated at a lower dose level, 0.06 mg/day, also showed improvement in swimming performance but not as much as those at the higher ginseng dose level of 0.6

mg/day. The data on swimming tests thus collect are listed in the following table. The table may give you a better understanding of the improved swimming performance of the ginseng treated mice over the controls.

Comparison of Swimming Performance of Mice at $18 \pm 0.1^{0}C.$*

	Group	Test	Mean Swimming Time, Secs.	Performance, % Improvement/control
1.	Control	First	476 ± 92	—
		Second	545 ± 121	—
2.	0.06 mg.-14 day	First	502 ± 97	5.4%
		Second	594 ± 133	9.0%
3.	0.6 mg.-14 day	First	582 ± 100	22.0%
		Second	610 ± 122	12.0%
4.	Control	First	496 ± 86	—
		Second	536 ± 83	—
5.	0.06 mg.-21 day	First	592 ± 104	19.5%
		Second	654 ± 140	22.0%
6.	0.6 mg.-21 day	First	630 ± 133	27.0%
		Second	645 ± 137	20.2%
7.	Control	First	466 ± 82	—
		Second	518 ± 96	—
8.	0.06 mg.-28 day	First	701 ± 130	51.8%
		Second	719 ± 134	38.8%
9.	0.6 mg.-28 day	First	668 ± 139	47.9%
		Second	717 ± 132	38.4%

*Each mouse was treated (except the control group) with ginseng extract, Geriatric Pharmaton, at levels of 0.06 or 0.6 mg. per mouse for 14, 21, and 28 days, respectively.

Using a similar procedure, Dr. Rueckert by using one thousand mice repeated the swimming study again in 1975. These mice were numbered and divided into several groups with fifty mice (twenty-five female and twenty-five male of similar body weight of about twenty grams) in each group. For each of the treated groups there was a separate control group of fifty mice, which were kept under the same conditions. They were allowed to swim at $18 \pm 0.1^{0}C$ until complete exhaustion, and the swimming time of each mouse was registered. After the first test, a dry-resting period of one hour was allowed, and then the mice were tested again (second test). Before the swimming experiment was conducted, the mice were treated (except the control group) with ginseng extract G-115 at 0.06 mg/day/mouse for, respectively, fourteen, twenty-one, and twenty-eight days. The controls were treated with placebo (water) daily. The results showed that mice treated with ginseng extract for fourteen days had about 5.1% increase in swimming performance at the first test and about 9.0% at the

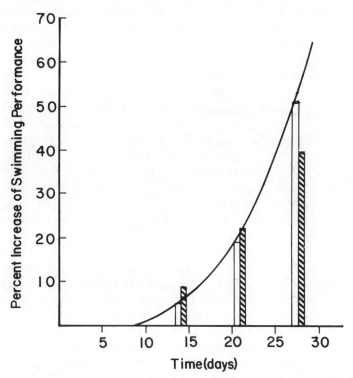

Shows the Increase in Swimming Performance in Mice Treated with Ginseng Extract, Geriatric Pharmaton G 115. The Percent of Increase is obtained by *Subtracting* the Mean Control Time from the Swimming Time of Mice Treated with Ginseng, *Divided* by the Mean Swimming Time of the Control, *Multiplied* by 100.

second test over the controls. After twenty-one days of treatment, the swimming improvements were about twenty percent at the first test and about twenty-two percent better at the second test over the controls. After twenty-eight days of treatment, however, the improvement was even more pronounced, about fifty two percent at the first test and about thirty-nine percent at the second test over the control group. These numbers are plotted in the figure below. The figure dipicts the percentage increase in swimming performance of mice after treatment with 0.06 mg/mouse/day of ginseng preparation (ginseng extract G-115) for fourteen, twenty-one, and twenty-eight days over the control mice. As a matter of fact, the curve clearly indicates that a much better improvement of swimming performance, called duration, was obtained after a relatively longer ginseng treatment.[11]

In a separate study, mice treated with two other ginseng extract preparations of two foreign companies, X-2 and S-II, for twenty-eight days, also showed some improvement in swimming performance over the controls. It seems that ginseng extract is indeed capable of improving the physical activities of animals, and the improvement could be reached at a relatively low dose. The biggest problem in this type of experiment would be the purity and strength of the ginseng preparation. In order to obtain dependable and reproduceable results, a standardized product has to be used.[11]

The antifatigue activity of ginseng extract was also investigated by the well-known Japanese pharmacologists Drs. H. Saito, M. Nabata, and K. Takagi of the University of Tokyo. In their studies, six different testing methods, e.g., exploratory movement, hole cross, rotating rod, sliding angle, spring balance, and rectal temperature tests were used. They evaluated the effect on different fractions of ginseng root extract on recovery from exhaustion. Four hours of oscillation exercise were used to exhaust the mice. Aqueous extracts of ginseng were injected intraperitoneally immediately following the exercise. It was observed that a water extract of ginseng significantly accelerated the recovery of exploratory movement and elevated rectal temperature. The antifatigue effect of a ginseng saponin, ginsenoside R_{g-1} and the lipophilic fraction of ginseng extract was more pronounced and more obvious in every test than that of other fractions isolated by the Japanese investigators.[12,13]

The swimming and running data clearly suggest that ginseng's antifatigue effect in mice may be also applicable to other animals and to humans for athletics or sports.[14] Quite interesting results were shown with horseracing in Japan and Korea back in the early twentieth century (Chapter 3). Recently a study with ginseng extract (Geriatric Pharmaton, G115) in forty-two sportsmen was conducted with a physical education unit in Liverpool, England, last year. These forty-two students had to undergo a training program with continuous medical checkups. This particular study showed that the sportsmen's stroke volume and cardiac output, reaction time, and respiratory quotient were significantly increased; in other words, the athletic performance, in general, was improved.[11] Having such a promising effect, the number of athletes from the Communist countries treated with ginseng tonic before attending the Olympic games is unknown.

Not too long ago, vitamin E, a modern chemical agent, had been claimed to prevent, among other things, ulcers, baldness, arthritis, diabetes, liver dysfunction, sexual impotence, and aging. The same vitamin has been recently added to cosmetics and used as a deodorant. Other claims have suggested that large doses of vitamin E can improve athletic performance;[15] however, in controlled trials, the E vitamin did not enhance the endurance of competitive swimmers.[16,17,18] The likelihood of serious adverse effects of vitamin E from such self-medication appears to be very low. Nevertheless, diarrhea and intestinal cramps have been reported with daily dose of 3200 IU of vitamin E.[18]

The antifatigue mechanism observed with ginseng and how it improves physical performance have been the subject of argument between Soviet and Chinese investigators. The Russian scientists, particularly Dr. Brekhman's group, are saying that ginseng basically is a "stimulant," and it has a marked stimulant effect.[19] On the contrary, based on their experiments the Chinese investigators, Dr. Tsung, *et al.*, of Kirin Medical Institute, proclaimed that the antifatigue activity of ginseng has a "sedative" instead of a "stimulant" effect.[20] The antifatigue action of ginseng was shown by the fact that the treated animals (rats) decreased their oxygen consumption, thus reducing the unnecessary tension and muscle exercise and fatigue, and their survival in a low-pressure (190/Hg.) chamber was also prolonged. This was confirmed with three experiments. In a mice swimming test, the swimming duration time of mice in the control group was 60 ± 10 minutes; the time for the ginseng-treated group, 88 ± 8 minutes (about 30 percent better than the control group); while the time for the caffeine-treated group was 47 ± 3 minutes. In another experiment, the mice were kept in reduced-pressure chambers. None of the ginseng-treated mice were dead, ten of twenty mice injected with sodium bromide were dead, and all of the twenty mice injected with caffeine were dead. A third experiment was the oxygen-consumption tests. It was found that the least oxygen was consumed after the injection of ginseng, in comparison with the amount consumed after injection of sodium bromide and chloropromazine, and the caffeine group showed the highest oxygen consumption.

Scicenkov studied the effect of ginseng on the visual performance of healthy young men. He found that, after a single administration of the liquid extracts of ginseng roots, the process of dark adaptation was accelerated, its final level was increased, and visual acuity also increased substantially. This may also be considered to be a tonic effect.[21]

It is an undisputable fact that ginseng can be considered as a tonic, a "safe" tonic. As Dr. Brekhman proclaimed about ginseng, "It possesses the stimulant action of other commonly used stimulants, but its safety is unique. It decreases a person's fatigue and boosts a person's working capacity as well as efficiency."[1] In clinical pharmacological tests, the tonic effect of ginseng on humans becomes apparent after both single and repeated doses. The tonic effect was observed not only during the treatment, but also three to four months later. The general tonic effects observed during the course of treatment with ginseng are: good mood, good appetite, good sleep, and absence of depressed state. Ginseng's tonic effect on animal organisms (including man) certainly has been proved.[6]

Enough evidence leads us to believe that excessive smoking causes lung cancer. The risk of dying from lung cancer for those who have smoked heavily for years is about twenty times greater than for nonsmokers.[26]

Breast cancer is also increasing and occurring in a younger age group than before. At least one in every twenty women in the United Kingdom was found to be suffering from breast cancer.[27]

Cancer may also be induced by psychological or nervous stress, particularly in women. "There is some casual link between cancer and the feeling of hopelessness, helplessness, despair, and depression," said Dr. James P. Henry, Professor of Physiology at the University of Southern California School of Medicine. Dr. Henry has paid a great deal of attention to studying why his laboratory female animals get breast tumors. He thinks the cause is despair, not rage, as when female mice are separated from their young.[28]

CAN GINSENG PREVENT CANCER?

Modern medical science still does not know how the change from a normal to an abnormal cell takes place. This is the main riddle of cancer. Certainly you are aware that noxious chemical fumes, polluted air and water, excessive cigarette smoking, excessive exposure to radiation, certain food dyes, food preservatives, food additives, and certain pesticides are possible carcinogens — agents that cause cancer.[22] With the advancement of the chemical and drug industries, new chemicals and drugs are placed on the market every day. More new synthetic drugs and chemicals introduced on the market mean more potential carcinogens.

In the United States, the cancer incidence is increasing steadily. In 1973, 37,000 persons died from colon and rectal cancer, 14,700 from stomach cancer, and 6,400 from esophogeal cancer.[23] The American Cancer Society estimated the death toll in 1974 to be 355,000, almost seventy-seven times the 46,181 American victims of combat in Vietnam, and 59,000 more than the 295,867 Americans who died on the battlefields during World War II.[24]

Aging is an important determinant of the incidence of cancer. Regardless of what the cancer may be, about one man in fourteen of those sixty years of age or older, as compared to one in seven hundred of those twenty-five or younger will develop cancer.[25]

Scientists have been desperately searching for anticancer drugs for years. Those available to date that act on gastrointestinal tract malignant tumors are: mitomycin, carmustine (BCNU), lumustine (CCNU), fluorouracil, fluorometholone, thiotepa, and nitrosourea. These potent chemotherapeutic agents have demonstrated some tumor inhibiting effect, yet none of them have shown outstanding success in the treatment of cancer.[29]

Russian scientists have devoted enormous time to ginseng research in the area of cancer prevention, if not treatment, in the past twenty-five years. In experimental oncology, ginseng preparations were capable of inihibiting urethane-induced adenomas of the lung, 6-methyl-thiouracil-induced tumors of the thyroid gland, and indole-induced myeloid leukemia in animals.[30,31,32] Cells of Ehrlich's ascitic tumor were introduced intravenously into mice, and ginseng exerted an effect of decreasing the transplantability and the size of tumorous foci.[33] Evidence was also obtained in the decrease of formation of spontaneous tumors of the mammary gland,[34] and spontaneous leukemia in mice.[35] Ether and alcoholic extracts of ginseng had a much greater effect than the aqueous extract in inhibiting malignant tumors in the secretory glands. However, ginseng had no effect on leukemia-1210 tumors.[36] With these preliminary findings, the use of ginseng or its components in the prevention of cancer may be possible in the future.

IMPOTENCE AND THE APHRODISIAC ACTIVITY OF GINSENG

Impotence is the most common sexual disability after forty-five years of age. Sexual failure is a serious problem; it can cause serious distress or uneasiness,[37] and it may precipitate an emotional crisis in a man that may threaten his life and his marriage.[38]

Factors Causing Male Impotence
- Psychogenic — 90% is due to psychologic factors
- Organic diseases — debilitating diseases
- Fatigue
- Intoxication with alcohols, drugs, and marijuana

Most sexual disorders including male impotence are mainly psychological in origin. However, even if you experience impotence, you may well still be able to attain an erection and function sexually under certain circumstances, for example, with a partner who knows how to make love, or with the help of a sexual stimulant remedy,[38,39] but most important of all, you must forget all your troubles and concentrate on love-making. Impotence may also be a consequence of organic disease. About half of all male diabetics become impotent before the age of 60.[39] Fatigue is another important factor leading to impotency. The husband, exhausted by his day's work, loses interest in love when he gets home; he may be over-dedicated to his job or his profession; his wife thinks he is married to his job, not to her. Besides physical fatigue, mental fatigue due to job difficulties, economic crisis, and depression may also be factors causing male impotence.

Statistically, heavy alcohol drinking is a common factor in impotence.[40] Marijuana, on the other hand, interferes with production of sexual hormones, in certain cases suppressing the male sex hormone, testosterone, to levels that could result in impotence and even infertility.[41]

There is no actual age limit for having or not having sex. There are thirty-year-old men who are inactive, and there are ninety-year-old men who still have active sex lives. Those leading a vigorous sex life in younger years tend to remain active longer. Good health, overall satisfaction with life, and the availability of a sanctioned sexual partner help maintain sexual activity's significant role in the life of the elder person.[42,43] At age sixty-eight, about seventy-eight percent of men still engage regularly in sexual activity. There are studies that have reported that sex around the age of ninety or one hundred is nothing unusual if a person is healthy and physically fit.[44]

Aphrodisiac Remedies All through history, people have searched for some means of revitalizing weakening sexual potency.

All kinds of treatments from all over the world have been tried, without notable success. Today, scientists finally may be on the trail of an authentic aphrodisiac. Several substances have shown attractive properties and may be useful as sexual stimulants for those who are impotent, particularly the aged.[45]

Many popular magazines carry advertisements advocating the use of oral preparations, sprays, and ointments for the genitalia that will increase sexual potency. The ingredients of these sexually stimulating preparations usually include vitamin E, whose role is quite unproved, together with varying mixtures of minerals and trace elements, carbohydrates, and proteins. Few of the preparations have any proven pharmacological effect.[46]

Spanish fly and yohimbine are some of the most well-known traditional aphrodisiacs.[45] Spanish fly is also called cantharides, or blistering fly. It is obtained from iridescent beetles found in southern France and Spain, and is an extremely harsh irritant. When swallowed in liquid form, it burns the mouth mucous membranes. According to Dr. Kent, the irritating effect of spanish fly can cause dilation of the blood vessels of the genital organs, leading to erection of the penis or congestion of the labia. Rather than being pleasurable, such physical arousal is unpleasant and dangerous. It causes gastroenteritis and nephritis. In fact, a large dose of spanish fly can be fatal. Yohimbine is a powder made from the inner bark of African yohimbe tree. It acts similarly on the blood vessels, but its aphrodisiac effect has been questionable.[45]

Parachlorophenylalanine (PCPA) is a chemical that can produce aphrodisiac effect in rats. However, PCPA is a very dangerous chemical that causes convulsions and other negative reactions. As a result, it has not been tested in humans.[45]

Some people who tout marijuana as having an aphrodisiac capacity contend that they enjoy sexual relations more when under influence of this perception-distorting drug. However, it has been proved that the sexual-stimulating effect of marijuana is similar to that of alcohol.[45]

Levodopa has been used extensively in humans, and has produced significant hypersexual behavior in man when it was administer for the treatment of Parkinson's disease.[47] There is controversy about the use of androgen (male sex hormone), however, and in most cases it found useless in the treatment of impotence.[48]

Ginseng's Aphrodisiac Action The great popularity of ginseng is probably based on its aphrodisiac activity. The reputed power of ginseng as an aphrodisiac has attracted the attention of millions of people.

Perhaps Dr. Eiberhof was the first Western scientist who tested the active principles from ginseng (panaquilon) in patients and found it exerts some aphrodisiac action.[49] Abe and Saito reported that ginsenin was active as an aphrodisiac and general mild stimulant to the sympathomimetic system.[50] Min found that ginsenin produced a tail erection effect in mice that maybe related to aphrodisiac properties.[51] Panax acid obtained from an ether extract of ginseng also produced a tail erection in mice.[52] The extracts from *P. ginseng* exhibited a greater activity than that from American ginseng in producing the tail erection effect in animals.[51]

The book *Ninjinshi (History of Ginseng)* written by T. Imamura, recorded that in the 1930s many Japanese and Korean hospitals used ginseng extracts in the treatment of impotence and some female sexual disorders.[53]

Some recent scientific investigators have provided more evidence for the gonadotropic or aphrodisiac action of ginseng. One study showed that ginseng has estrogenic properties.[54] In experiments with animals, a gonadotropic effect of ginseng was established as manifested by causing infantile male and female mice to reach puberty earlier than they would have otherwise. The gonadotropic activities of ginseng saponins, panaxosides A, C, D, E, and F, exerted a similar, but stronger effect than that of crude ginseng extract. However Kit[55] and Wang[56] reported that ginseng does not possess any male or female sex hormone activity, based on the fact that administration of ginseng preparations could not restore the castrated male and ovarilectomized female animals to normal. However, ginseng contains certain principles that do stimulate and promote an animal's sexual maturity.

Ginseng was given orally to (normal) rats in a daily dose of 0.1-0.2 g. for sixty one days, or the rats were injected with 10 mg. of methanol extract of ginseng for eight days. There was no remarkable change in growth of either female or male rats, nor was any change observed in the sexual cycle between experimental and control rats.[57]

Whether or not the active principles of ginseng root contain any sex hormone activity has been puzzling for a long time, and only a few reports are aviailable to date. Female hormonelike activity was observed in one study after a methanol extract of ginseng was given to female mice.[58] By a thin-layer chromatographic technique, estrogen-type (female hormone) components of estrone, estradiol, and estriol were isolated from an oil-soluble fraction of ginseng extract.[59] This is the first time that ginseng was found to contain sex hormones or sex hormonelike substances.

Using a biochemical approach, it was found that an alcoholic extract of ginseng increased the testicular RNA and DNA levels of rats. Professor Oura and associates observed in a series of investigations that ginseng extracts, particularly fraction number four, increased the synthesis of DNA and protein in test tubes. It is assumed that the synthesis of RNA and protein may be equally promoted in the testes.[60,61,62]

In another recent experiment using mesenteric mast cells as indicators, it was found that ginseng preparations have the ability to increase the number of mast cells. In the castrated male rat, ginseng functions like testosterone by decreasing the deterioration of the mast cells.[62]

Recent clinical studies in humans in Japan and in the Soviet Union show that ginseng extract was quite effective toward several forms of impotence, particularly the premature ejaculation-type impotence and nervous-type impotence. It is not effective for psychic-type impotence.[56] The aphrodisiac activity of ginseng seemed to be proven correct. As a sexual tonic, ginseng is probably the safest aphrodisiac agent in comparison with all other chemicals speculated around the world.

QUIETING YOUR SPIRIT

The central nervous system is the most highly organized of all the systems of the body. It may be considered as being superimposed upon all other organs for the purpose of coordinating their diverse functions toward a harmonious functioning of the organism as a whole. Because of its complex structure, delicate ramifications, and supreme importance to the body, the central nervous system is extremely sensitive to all drugs. How does ginseng affect the central nervous system? This problem has been the number-one research project, and a dozen of the top pharmacologists in the world have investigated it.

The pharmacological properties of ginseng claimed in the earliest Chinese materia medica books as:

> "quieting the spirit, establishing the soul,
> allaying fear, brightening the eyes,
> benefiting the understanding. . .,"

are a beautiful and factual description of ginseng's activities on the central nervous system. How did the Chinese doctors know all about this even two thousand years ago? Only after fifty years of scientific research has it been proved that the activities of ginseng on the central nervous system (CNS) are its principle pharmacological properties. Also, ginseng's activities on the CNS are most confusing.[6]

The early pharmacological studies on ginseng in Japan revealed the rather complex effect of ginseng's properties on the nervous system. For example, Fujitani found that panaquilon has hypnotic and depressant activities.[63] Panax acis and panacene similarly showed weak sedative and hypnotic effects on the cerebral centers, but they stimulated the vasomotor and respiratory centers, thus increasing blood flow and pressure and the rate of respiration when given in small doses, but lowering the blood pressure when given in large doses.[64,65,66] Yonekawa[67] investigated the various pharmacological activities of ginsenin. A stimulant effect on the nervous system in mice was observed using small doses, and a depressant effect was obtained using large doses. Ginseng saponins (extracted from ginseng roots) had stimulatory effects on the central nervous system (CNS) in rats, as was shown by decreased sleeping components and increased activity components.[68] Ginseng saponins increased in low doses(2.5-5.0 mg/kg.), but decreased in high doses (100 mg/kg.), the spontaneous motor activity in mice and rats.[69] Apparently in small doses, ginseng saponins stimulate the central nervous system, but the mode of action is different from that of amphetamine or benzedrinelike compounds.[70] The stimulant action of ginseng is characterized by low toxicity, absence of pronounced excitation, and lack of disturbance of normal sleep. Ginseng is a remedy having few side-effects in comparison to other known chemical stimulants.[1]

Again, from the studies of ginseng aqueous extract, the Chinese scientists found that ginseng was a potent sedative.[20] It weakens respiratory systems, slows spontaneous activity, and also prevents the convulsion provoked by a number of central nervous stimulants, such as caffeine, sodium benzoate, strychnine nitrate, and cardiazol (pentalenetetrazole).

Recently, Professor Tagaki and his associates at the Faculty of Pharmaceutical Sciences, University of Tokyo, conducted a series of systemic pharmacological studies on ginseng extracts and ginseng saponins.[71,72] The crude ginseng extract was separated into several fractions, and each fraction contained two to three individual saponins. The first fraction (G No. 3, containing ginsenosides R_b and R_c) showed central nervous system depressive, ataractic, analgesic, and muscle-relaxant activities in mice, rats, and guinea pigs. The second fraction (G No. 4 containing ginsenosides $R_{g\text{-}1}$, $R_{g\text{-}2}$ and $R_{g\text{-}3}$) had both stimulant and depressant activities, in addition to muscarinic and histaminic actions. The third fraction (G No.5 containing lipophilic saponins) had papaverinelike in addition to muscarinic and histaminic actions. Fractions No. 4 and No. 5 had central depressant action such as decreased spontaneous movement, decreased body temperature and alertness, and relaxed muscle tone. Accordingly, ginsenosides of the protopanaxadiol series (R_b group) are sedatives, while ginsenosides of the protopanaxatriol series R_g group are mostly stimulants. This explains why ginseng extract contains both *depressant* and *stimulant* components.[72] Dr. Kaku *et al.* further investigated the pharmacological properties of each of the individual purified ginseng saponins, $R_{b\text{-}1}$, $R_{b\text{-}2}$, R_c, R_d, R_e, R_f, $R_{g\text{-}1}$, and $R_{g\text{-}2}$. Their data show that all the saponins exhibited antifatigue action. They markedly increased the movement after compulsory gait, and the action was consistent and independent of their action on the movement before compulsory gait. These saponins also showed moderate depressant actions on the EEG and in the behavior of cats. Saponins R_{g-1}, R_e, and R_{b-2} are more potent than the others.[73]

Many clinical tests in the Soviet Union in the early 1950s revealed that ginseng extracts are effective for patients who are suffering from different types of nervous exhaustion and several emotional disorders.[1,74] After treatment with ginseng, the patients showed weight gain with the disappearance of common symptoms such as weakness, fatigue, headache, insomnia, distress, and uneasiness. Ginseng extract also produced good results in a number of other emotional disorders such as mental weakness and exhaustion, various emotional disorders including vegitative nervous disorders, hypertension, gonadal disorders, hypotension, and loss of appetite. It seems from clinical experience that ginseng extract would be useful as a supplementary remedy for emotional disorders.[74]

IMPROVING MENTAL EFFICIENCY AND WORKING CAPACITY

The influence of ginseng on working capacity and mental efficiency is a new dimension of pharmacological research. That ginseng increases memory has been claimed by the ancient Chinese doctors. According to Dr. Brekhman, however, "The fact that ginseng increases both mental capacity and quantitative indices of work in laboratories and at industrial occupations indicates its powerful effect upon a specific portion of the central nervous system." It was assumed that ginseng may have a particular and, most probably, electrical effect on the highest sections of the central nervous system.[6] Ginseng has a favorable effect on the cerebral cortex process, and makes the conditioned reflexes easier, thus ginseng is capable of increasing the mental efficiency of man.

Many studies have been conducted in the Soviet Union and in Sweden to prove that ginseng increases mental efficiency. In proof-reading, all the tests showed that ginseng helped to lessen the number of mistakes (by about 51%), while the number of letters read was only slightly increased (by about 12%). Ginseng extract was also tested in telegraph operators who had to transcribe a special code in a fixed period of time. Ordinarily, the continued work would result in an increase in the number of errors of about 128%, while in the operators who took 30 ml. of ginseng extract, the number of mistakes decreased by about 38%.[6]

In a recent study in Stockholm, healthy college students served as volunteers in a double-blind experiment lasting for thirty-three days. The volunteers were divided into three groups, each group containing five male and five female students. The students were treated with two ginseng capsules per day. The tests conducted were the spiral maze test and the letter cancellation test. At the end of the thirty-three day tests, the students given ginseng extract (Geriatric-Pharmaton or Gerikomplex-Vitamex)* treatment had fewer errors than the control group who were treated with placebo capsules. Also it was found that the two ginseng preparations exerted an almost equally favorable effect on psychomotor function and on the mental capacity. In other words, students given ginseng showed a statistically significant increase in mental concentration.[75]

Accordingly, a healthy individual may increase his capacity for intellectual work in addition to physical performance under the influence of ginseng. The improvement of work is qualitative but not quantitative; in this regard, ginseng may increase industrial productivity. This is, as Dr. Brekhman called it, "the tonic effect on man's organism" to prove that ginseng is a remedy that when taken for some time, causes increased vitality, leading to greater work efficiency and mental capacity.

REGULATING YOUR BLOOD PRESSURE

Hypertension is one of the most common human disorders and a major cause of complications leading to death in middle-

*Geriatric—pharmaton and Gerikomplex—vitamex are ginseng-vitamin preparations of Pharmaton, Ltd. Lugano, Switzerland.

aged and aged individuals. At least twenty-three million people in the United States have hypertension, which is a major risk factor for strokes and heart failure. There is a substantial increase in hypertensive heart disease with age in both sexes. Blacks have substantially more heart diseases and hypertension than whites, and usually males have more than females.

How Ginseng Acts on the Cardiovascular System Although it is premature to say that ginseng is effective in its treatment or prevention of hypertensive or hypotensive heart diseases, the effects of ginseng on the heart, blood pressure, blood vessels, and even respiratory systems are medically significant. Quite a number of studies have been reported in medical literature. The sedative effect of ginseng, i.e., lowering the blood pressure, has been the most interesting and pharmacologically useful observation.

Yonekawa[67] observed that ginsenin increased the function of an isolated frog's heart at a small dose, but paralyzed it at a large dose. Kin[52] found similar effects with panax acid. In studies with nonisolated hearts of frogs and cats, ginseng showed similar dose-dependent stimulant-depressant effects. In other studies, ginsenin,[67] panaquilon,[63] and panax acid[65,66] all showed blood pressure lowering (depressor) but not pressure increasing effects in animals. Kin[52] and Watanabe,[76] on the other hand, reported that ginseng and ginseng saponin caused an increase in blood pressure (pressure effect) at small doses, but a pressure lowering (depressor effect), which remained for some time, occurs at large doses in rabbits. Injection of ginseng extract also caused a depressor effect in the anesthetized dogs.[77]

Toward the blood vessels, the alcoholic extract of ginseng initially contracts, then dilates, the capillary blood vessels in frogs. Ginsenin showed a vasocontraction effect in frogs and rabbits at small doses, but a vasodilation effect was observed at large doses.[67]

Administration of ginseng saponins, ginsenosides, to dogs caused a remarkable increase in blood flow, and the effect was more potent than that induced by papaverine. Ginsenosides also showed a vasodilator effect. The ginsenoside R_{g-1} at a dose of 5 to 10 mg/kg. had a depressor effect preceeded by a slight pressor effect, but the respiration was little affected. The dose-dependent raising-lowering of blood pressure (biphasic effect) seemed to be due to the direct action of the ginseng saponin on the blood vessels.[73] Because of the vasodilation effect of the capillary vessels, ginseng extract also increased the blood supply to tissues and the brain.[78]

The depressor effect, as a matter of fact, has been adopted in China as well as in the Soviet Union as an indicator in biological analysis for potency determination of ginseng preparations.[56] In other words, the potency of a ginseng preparation can thus be standardized. The practical application of the depressor effect in humans after an oral dose of ginseng, however, is still questionable and more research definitely is needed to prove it.

Other studies in China showed that ginseng has direct dynamic action on the blood flow, with an increase in the force of cardiac contraction, especially during acute circulatory failure or shock.[79] The effect of ginseng in normalizing the level of arterial pressure is indeed unique. It is effective in the treatment of abnormal hypotension. Clinical research conducted at Hwa-san Hospital in Shanghai showed interesting results. In seven cases of acute interference with blood flow of the heart muscle (myocardial infarction) with shock irregularity in the rhythm of the heart's beating. The patients were treated by a routine method or with ginseng. When a Western type of drug was given to raise the blood pressure, the blood pressure rose only temporarily, then fell in a short time even after repeated doses. However, when ginseng preparations, either alone or in conjunction with *seng fu tang,** were given to similar patients, the blood pressure rose and remained at a normal level. In addition ginseng also prevented shock, and patients returned to normal.[80]

GINSENG CONTROLS BODY'S
CHOLESTEROL AND ATHEROSCLEROSIS

Cholesterol is produced naturally in our body and exists in blood, bile, and the gallbladder. Another direct source of

---

Seng fu tang — a mixture made by decocting ginseng, 15.6 g. and *fu-tze* (Aconitum carmichaeli D.) 12.48 g. to a thick liquid.

cholesterol is foods such as beef drippings, milk, eggs, cheese, butter, cream, organ meats, etc., all of which contain high levels of cholesterol.

The cholesterol content in blood is usually maintained at a constant level. For example, if dietary sources are high in cholesterol, less cholesterol will be formed in the liver. A number of hormones markedly affect the formation of cholesterol and its degradation. For example, insulin and thyroid hormone deficient people usually suffer from high cholesterol.

According to Drs. T. Dawber and Kannel of the Framingham Heart study, a man under fifty-nine with a blood cholesterol measurement of 260 or above has more than three times the risk of heart attack than a man with a blood cholesterol level below 200.

Laboratory testing animals—monkeys, dogs, cats, pigs, chickens, rats, guinea pigs, and hamsters—fed a high-fat and high-cholesterol diet, developed atherosclerosis and heart attacks, resulting in deaths sooner, and in more instances, than in those fed with a low cholesterol diet. This is similar to what is observed with humans.

At present, atherosclerosis, particularly of the coronary arteries, is the most widespread illness in the United States. In 1965, nearly forty percent of all deaths in the United States were due to heart attacks caused by atherosclerosis. Of these deaths, nearly one-third occurred in people under the age of sixty-five. Today, about one in five American males will develop coronary disease before the age of sixty. The chance that he will die of the heart disease before sixty is about one in fifteen.[81]

If you have high blood cholesterol, your doctor may have told you to eat a low cholesterol and low fat diet. You may have known that in order to reduce cholesterol in the diet you have to use unsaturated vegetable oils for cooking, instead of saturated oil, animal fat, butter, or lard; switch from deep-fried foods to boiled foods; eat less cheese, milk, egg yolk, liver, and butter. You may also want to switch from regular cheese to cottage cheese, whole milk to skim milk or even soybean milk, and eat more fish, chicken, and turkey instead of beef, pork, duck and bacon. You may even want to cut your regular

American diet with Chinese dishes, which contain less cholesterol and less calories.

Ginseng Controls Cholesterol Level From animal studies, ginseng saponins show a marked effect on the regulation of blood cholesterol levels. After administration of ginseng, animals showed an increase in the synthesis of cholesterol in the liver, but the total cholesterol concentration in the serum decreased by about twenty-five percent, as a result of decreased absorption of cholesterol from the gastrointestinal tract and also an increase in the speed of cholesterol metabolism in the animal's body. In addition abnormal (high) cholesterol levels in the blood and deposit of fat in the heart can be prevented when ginseng is included in the diet.[82]

The effect of ginseng on blood cholesterol levels in connection with diet and antisclerotic drugs was investigated. Dr. Popov of the Revitalization Center at Nassau, Bahamas, found that with ginseng preparations in combination with antisclerotic drugs, the cholesterol levels of the blood fell nearly twenty percent, in the treatment of 106 patients aged from forty to seventy years, suffering from hypertension and high blood cholesterol. Dr. Popov concluded that ginseng extract possesses a substantial synergistic effect in reducing blood cholesterol concentration.[83]

ANTIDIABETIC EFFECT OF GINSENG

Diabetes is a universal disease that is encountered most frequently in industrialized countries, particularly among poor and older people. Despite the important medical advances in the treatment of the disease and its complications, diabetes has accounted for about 38,000 deaths a year in the United States since 1965, and has been implicated as a contributory cause in a substantial proportion of deaths from other chronic diseases. Diabetes has been characterized by consistently higher mortality rate among females than among males.[84] It is more interesting to note that, from 1964 to 1973, the mortality rate from diabetes among men insured under standard, ordinary policies of the Metropolitan Life Insurance Company decreased by twenty percent, while that among insured women increased by five percent. Diabetes has become the nation's third-ranking cause of death, behind cardiovascular disease and cancer, and is increasing rapidly at a rate of about one million new diabetics every three years. The disease is about three times as common among the poor as among the middle-income families and the rich.

In diabetes the metabolism of carbohydrates is impaired, and that of proteins and fats is enhanced. Glucose in the body thus builds up to high levels, especially in the blood (hyperglycemia), and is excreted in the urine (glucosuria). The breakdown of tissue proteins, lipids, and fatty acids is sharply accelerated in diabetics, thus producing a large amount of nitrogen and ketone bodies in the urine. The excretion of glucose and ketone bodies causes a big loss of body water and salt, thus producing a dehydration effect and a feeling of great thirst. In severe cases, it can produce ketoacidosis (a disease of high ketone in the urine), coma, and eventually death, if the condition is not corrected by the administration of insulin.

Obesity is the most common contributing factor to diabetes. Heredity also appears to be an important factor. The life expectancy of diabetics is estimated to be shorter by one-third than that of nondiabetics. Failure to control the diabetic state may lead to serious complications. Cataracts and blindness, leg gangrene, heart disorders, including atherosclerosis, and kidney failure are the most common diabetic complications. Diabetes is also the second leading cause of blindness in the United States.

Drugs lowering the blood sugar level are called hypoglycemics. Insulin had been the most effective anti-diabetic drug. However, it is ineffective orally. Unfortunately most of the clinically available oral hypoglycemic drugs have undersirable side effects. Recent research findings show that treatment of diabetes with oral hypoglycemic drugs may be associated with increased rate of cardiovascular mortality, when compared to the treatment of diabetes with diet alone or diet plus insulin.[85] The effect of ginseng on hyperglycemia has been extensively investigated both at laboratory and clinical levels. Preliminary data showed promising and interesting.

Ginseng for Diabetes One of the most important medicinal uses of ginseng is its activity for diabetic patient. Ginseng's activity toward diabetes seemed to be known to Chinese doctors as early as the first century. Dr. T'ao, Hung-ching's *Ming-I Pieh-lu,* a famous Chinese medical book published before the Han dynasty, described the usefulness of ginseng in eliminating tiredness, thirstiness, and polyurea, which are the most common symptoms of diabetes. Other famous Chinese medical compendium of the old days, such as *Hai-yao Pen-ts'ao* written by Li, Heng of T'ang dynasty, and *Yung-Yao-Fa Hsiang-lun* by Dr. Li, Tung-yuan of Yuan dynasty and *Pen-ts'ao Kang-mu,* edited by the most famous pharmacologist and physician, Li, Shih-chen of the Meng dynasty, recorded the uses of ginseng to relieve the ailment or symptoms related to diabetes.

There are at least twenty-five separate modern scientific studies of ginseng's activities in diabetes conducted in Japan, China, Bulgaria, the Soviet Union, and Korea. The pioneer Japanese workers in this area, Arima and Miyazaki,[86] who treated high blood sugar (hyperglycemia) in rabbits with ginseng saponin, observed, as with ginseng extract, a blood sugar lowering (hypoglycemic) effectg. Kin[87] reported that subcutaneous injection of ginseng saponin, panax acid (an active component of ginseng), or oral administration of panacene (another active component of ginseng) to rabbits, produced a marked hypoglycemic effect. Particularly, ginseng saponin inhibited adrenaline-induced hyperglycemia, but questionable results were obtained on hyperglycemia induced by ammonium chloride.

In China during the 1950s C. K. Wang and H. P. Lei of Peking University,[88,89] C. Y. Sung and T. H. Chen[90] of the Chinese Academy of Medical Sciences in Peking, and C. Tsuao and C. C. Yen[91,92] made separate studies on the effect of ginseng in alloxan diabetes. Their data, as were reported to the First Conference of the Society of Chinese Physiological Sciences in 1956, indicated that the application of ginseng extract decreased blood sugar and urine acetate in alloxan-induced hyperglycemia in dogs, rats, and mice. Later in 1957, Wang and Lei,[88] by using a ginseng preparation (a fifty percent alcohol extract of red-ginseng and dried) to normal and alloxan-induced diabetic male dogs. With daily doses of 0.13, 0.2, and 1.0 mg/kg of body weight, for two weeks, observed the hypolycemic effect of ginseng when given alone or in combination with protamine-zinc insulin. The average blood sugar levels in the period five to ten days prior to ginseng administration was compared with that during the last day of treatment. In the normal dogs, the administration of 1 mg/kg of ginseng preparation produced somewhat drops in the blood sugar levels. On the other hand, a dosage of 0.2 mg/kg produced no significant change, but in another dog it produced a rise in blood sugar level. In the diabetic dogs, the ginseng preparation at 1 mg/kg produced a significant decrease in blood sugar levels. Apparent falls in the urine output and urine sugar were sometimes observed during the treatment. Although the dose level of 0.2 mg/kg failed to change the blood sugar level, in every instance, the general condition and urine ketone reactions were improved during the period of ginseng treatment. In spite of the fact that ginseng had a hypoglycemic effect (at high doses) in the normal and diabetic animals, it was unable to completely correct the metabolic disturbance occurring in alloxan-diabetic dogs and, therefore, failed to check the diabetic state. It may be helpful in the treatment of the diabetic state, but it cannot be relied upon to act as a substitute for insulin.[56]

In 1959, Tsuao, Yen and Lei further reported that ginseng normalized blood sugar levels in alloxan-induced diabetic mice but did not prevent their death.[92] Liu, Chi, and Sung[93] studied the effect of ginseng on alloxan diabetes in rats fed different diets. In the first series of experiments, seventeen rats were divided into two groups and were given alloxan, 200 mg/kg, intraperitoneally. One group of the animals (six rats) was fed with cornmeal, a high carbohydrate diet, plus five percent of ginseng powder in the cornmeal, while the second group (eleven rats) was fed only with cornmeal for a total of twelve weeks (one week prior to and eleven weeks after the injection of alloxan). After three days of alloxan injection, three of the eleven rats in the control group were dead, while only one rat in the ginseng-fed group was dead. Of the remaining eight rats in the control group, six rats developed diabetes, the

THE EFFECT OF *P. GINSENG* ON ALLOXAN-DIABETES IN RATS FED WITH CORN MEAL

	RATS	Mean Serum Sugar Levels mg%										
WEEK		1	2	3	4	5	6	7	8	9	10	11
5% ginseng powder added in Diet	1	339	310	176	146	116	130	168	112	125	140	83
	2	600	600	589	600	584	364	160	128	245	214	190
	3	463	420	294	255	208	274	160	170	146	152	148
	4	197	174	128	139	148	160	144	141	175	130	102
	5	170	144	143	139	130	136	152	130	136	116	128
Control (No ginseng)	1	554	dead									
	2	585	dead									
	3	524	600	dead								
	4	600	600	dead								
	5	600	600	600	600	600	dead					
	6	600	600	576	600	600	600	dead				
	7	167	162	122	126	116	144	120	130	110	80	101
	8	222	198	145	143	152	176	162	130	140	124	101

Data after Liu, K-T, H.C. Chi and Shen-yu Sung
Acta Pharm. Sinica, 7: 213   (1959).

blood sugar levels were about 557 ± 17 mg%, and seven weeks later, all of the six diabetic rats were dead. In the ginseng-fed group, however, among the six rats, one was dead and three developed mild diabetes; the average blood sugar levels were 587 ± 75 mg%. The rats continued with five percent ginseng powder in the feed gradually lowered their blood sugar levels to normal and remained at normal blood sugar levels (ca. 150 mg%) for at least three weeks after the withdrawal of ginseng treatment. As shown in the following table, the alloxan-induced diabetic rats' high blood sugar levels reduced to normal seven weeks after the continued administration of five percent ginseng in the diet, while the diabetic rats of the control group were all dead within seven weeks.

In another series of experiments wherein the rats were fed a high-protein diet (a mixture of fish powder, beans, whole wheat, bone meal, yeast powder, and cod liver oil), the blood sugar levels of the alloxan-diabetic rats treated with ginseng did not differ significantly from those of the untreated diabetic rats. It appears that the *diet* of the animals made the results of the two series of experiments contradictory. Nevertheless, when the high-protein diet was replaced by cornmeal during the latter half of the experiment, the blood sugar levels of the untreated rats increased drastically while no significant change in blood sugar levels was observed in the ginseng-treated rats. This experiment clearly indicated that although the rats fed with five percent ginseng for one week could not escape the action of alloxan, ginseng, ultimately, did normalize the blood sugar levels of alloxan-induced diabetic rats, particularly when the rats were fed a high-carbohydrate diet.

Studies in the Soviet Union and Bulgaria in the 1950s and 1960s further supported the theme of ginseng's uses in diabetes. In the treatment of alloxan-induced diabetes ginseng was found to impede a loss of body weight of rats, to reduce the sugar levels in the urine, and to prolong the survival time of the diabetic animals.[94] Another study showed an extract of ginseng reduced the high blood sugar levels in rabbits with adrenaline hyperglycemia, and in humans with alimentary hyperglycemia.[95]

According to Petkov,[96] ginseng evidently is capable of potentiating the action of insulin. It is very surprising that ginseng extract regulates the carbohydrate metabolism both ways, i.e., in an experimentally induced hyperglycemic state, ginseng was able to reduce the blood sugar level, while in an insul-induced hypoglycemic state, ginseng could bring about an increase in the blood sugar level to normal.[97] Isn't it amazing?

From biochemical approaches, the effect of ginseng on carbohydrate metabolism has been evaluated by many investigators. Lee[98] found that ginseng may contain a substance that is capable of increasing the basal metabolism in normal rats, in this regard, the effects could be blocked by anti-histaminic agents. Based on this finding, it was believed that the effect of ginseng on metabolism may be due to histamine liberation, or that ginseng may stimulate the liberation of histamine in the body.

In 1973 Professors Oura and Hiai[99] of Toyama University reported that after intraperitoneal injection of ginseng extract (a fraction 4), the liver glycogen and the reducing sugar levels in rats were reduced. Ginseng saponin contained in the extract somehow caused a decrease in the total carbohydrate level in the animal. Ginseng extract caused a marked reduction in the blood glucose levels of rats with adrenal glands removed, but had a weak or insignificant effect in normally fed rats and in fasted rats infused with glucose solution. The reduction of blood sugar was observed two hours after the injection of ginseng, and this effect continued for about eight hours. Also, in rats, liver glycogen content and the sugar levels in the liver, kidney, and muscles were also remarkedly reduced after the treatment with ginseng extract.[100] The authors suggested that ginseng extract turns the metabolic flow in the direction of lipogensis by the conversion of sugar. This was confirmed by the fact that the first phenomenon observed was a striking stimulation in the incorporation of radio-activity into the adipose tissue beginning two hours after the administration of ginseng. Almost simultaneously a slight decrease of blood sugar level was also observed.[101] The investigators also found that the glycogen content of rat liver varies with diet. Similarly, from the application of an radio isotope, sodium ^{14}C-acetate, the incorporation of the ^{14}C-acetate into the total lipid and glycogen content in the liver was determined four hours after injection of ginseng extract into rats. The results indicated that a striking stimulation of metabolism was obtained in rats fed a fat-free diet over the high-fat diet group.[102]

The early clinical studies on the hypoglycemic effect of ginseng were conducted in Korea and Japan in the 1930s. In the treatment of diabetic patients, Saito[103] and Saito and Abe[104] found that the alcoholic extract of ginseng was effective in inhibiting adrenaline hyperglycemia and alimentary hyperglycemia. In Japanese hospitals in the early days, diabetic patients were treated with ginseng powder or by injection with ginseng extract. The blood sugar levels and the general symptoms of the diabetic patients were indeed reduced, but a cure of the diabetes was not obtained.

In the Soviet Union, Shass[105] reported that the treatment of diabetic patients with seventy percent alcoholic extract of ginseng gave good results and Dr. Shass even suggested that ginseng could substitute for insulin. The hypoglycemic effect was very good during winter and fall seasons, but not so good during the spring and summer seasons.

Recent clinical studies in China showed that ginseng was capable of lowering the blood sugar levels to about 40 to 50 mg% in diabetic patients. This hypoglycemic effect continued for about two weeks after the treatment. Unfortunately, ginseng, like other chemical hypoglycemic agents on the market, exerted no curative effect in moderate and severe diabetic patients; general symptoms such as thirst, weakness, and polyurea, however, were much improved, or disappeared. Ginseng cannot substitute for insulin; in patients who use insulin for treatment, the insulin dose level could be decreased if ginseng is concomitantly administered.[56]

During the period of January to July of 1970, Dr. T. Kikutani of Sanraku Hospital, Tokyo, investigated the effect of ginseng on diabetic patients clinically. Twenty-one diabetic outpatients (thirteen male and eight female) were the subjects, and they all complained of having common subjective symptoms of fatigue and malaise, hypertension, thirst, protein urea, increased intake of water, loss of energy, coldness, and lumbago. These patients were treated with a ginseng preparation in capsules (a commercial product of Yamanouchi Drug Co., Japan), one capsule each time, three capsules a day for four to six months. Each capsule contained 100 mg of dried, powdered ginseng extract and 20 mg of vitamin E. The blood sugar levels and other symptoms of the patients were examined periodically. From this pilot clinical study, it was found that the ginseng extract was effective on fifteen out of the eighteen diabetic patients. Their subjective symptoms were improved and their blood sugar levels were reduced to normal along with the treatment.[106]

In another clinical trial, Professors Y. Kakiochi, T. Imanaka, N. Kohuo, T. Ohara, and T. Nakajima of Osaka University, School of Medicine, treated eighteen diabetic patients with the same ginseng preparation as that used in the studies described above. However, in this study, the patients were allowed to take two capsules each time, three times a day, i.e., each patient takes 600 mg of ginseng extract and 120 mg of vitamin E per day. The duration of the treatment varied from fourteen to eighty four days depending upon the conditions of the patient. The patients were questioned about their symptoms regularly and their blood, stool, and urine samples were analyzed, and their renal and hepatic functions were checked by the staffs of the same hospital. The results showed that ginseng was effective in four out of seven patients against general malaise, three out of five patients against tiredness and fatigue, four out of five patients against impotence, and three out of three patients against thirst. In other words, the ginseng extract at 600 mg level daily dose was about 60 to 100% effective in the treatment of the subjective symptoms of the diabetic. Also found was that ginseng was able to improve the anemic conditions of the patient. In insulin-resistant patients, ginseng was able to reduce the dose level of insulin if ginseng was concomitantly used. The investigators also indicated that the 600 mg dose of ginseng may be required in the onset of the treatment, but a 300 mg maintenance dose may be sufficient for chronic patients who need a long-term therapy. In both of the studies, no particular reason was given why vitamin E was added in the ginseng capsules.[106]

THE REMARKABLE HEMATINIC EFFECT OF GINSENG

Anemia When the number of red blood cells or the amount of hemoglobin within them falls below certain levels, a person is said to have anemia. Anemia often causes pallor, weakness, wanness, lack of vigor, and most important of all, susceptibility to other diseases. Anemia patients have high mortality rate and, therefore, every effort should be taken to reduce or prevent its occurence.

The loss of a large amount of blood from the body (usually from a bleeding wound, bleeding from the gastrointestinal tract, an ulcer, or due to abnormal menstruation in women) may cause anemia. A drop in red blood cell production as a result of iron-deficiency in diet, malnutrition, organic diseases, or inability to absorb the bloodmaking elements such as vitamin B_{12}, folic acid, and iron may cause anemia. Degeneration, defectiveness, or short life of red blood cells may also induce anemia. Nevertheless, iron-deficiency is the most frequent cause of anemia.[107,108]

Ginseng's Hematinic Effect From animal studies, ginseng acts as a powerful hematinic agent. It increases hemoglobin levels and restores red blood cells quickly in animals after bleeding. Kin[109] observed that rabbits receiving 0.5 g/kg. daily of ginseng alcoholic extract showed a rapid increase in the number of red blood cells, which continued for about a month and then ceased. The hemoglobin content and the white blood cell (leukocyte) counts were also greatly increased. An hematinic iron preparation, Blutone (a strong antianemia agent), given at 13 g/kg. to rabbits as a control, induced a lesser increase in red blood cells and hemoglobin than did ginseng extract. Ginseng was thus called a hematinic. Several other studies showed ginseng causing an increase in the number of red blood cells and hemoglobin in animals.[110] Ginseng extract also showed fast restoration of blood albumin in animals after massive bleeding.[111]

Recently, a group of Japanese investigators, Professor Oura *et al.*, reported that intraperitoneal injection of ginseng extract to rats and mice increased the synthesis of serum proteins.[112,113,114] Serum proteins synthesis increased by about 46 to 49%. Ginseng extract also stimulated the synthesis of ribonucleic acid (RNA) in rat's liver, in addition to the synthesis of bone marrow deoxyribonucleic acid (DNA), and the normal division of bone marrow cells. The active principles of ginseng extract, particularly the ginsenosides, are expected to have a metabolic-stimulating or hormone-like action. Biochemical studies have added further positive evidence supporting the thesis that ginseng is a hematinic agent. Regarding the hematinic effect, one of the active principles of ginseng, *prostisol*, plays an essential role in protein and RNA synthesis in the rats' liver.[115,116]

The hematinic effect of ginseng was also demonstrated in humans, particularly those who have been ill for a long time, are suffering from wasteful or consumptive diseases, or are recovering from major surgery. Following surgical operations for gastric ulcer, patients in a Soviet hospital were given the conventional treatment and care, and a special group was given additional ginseng preparations. It was found that the patients treated with ginseng were the first restored to health and returned to work.[19] In a recent clinical trial at National Shirahama Hot Spring Hospital in Japan, the efficacy of an aqueous extract of ginseng (containing prostisol) on fatigue and anemia was critically evaluated. The ginseng extract was particularly effective in the treatment of anemia due to tuberculosis, old age, and iron-deficiency, but ineffective toward pernicious anemia. In addition, the symptoms associated with anemia, such as rheumatoid arthritis, fatigue, and debility, were eliminated. Appetite, hemoglobin level, and the number of red blood cells and platelets were greatly improved or increased. Among the fifty patients treated no one complained of any side-effect with ginseng.[117]

IMPROVEMENT OR CURE FOR INDIGESTION

When we say indigestion or digestive disorders, it means the digestive system may not be in the normal working order.

When digestion is so below par that the food remains un-digested, it causes the growth and multiplication of putrefac-tive bacteria—germs capable of decomposing of foods, resulting in the generation of foul gases. The most common in-digestion disturbance, particularly in the middle aged and the aged, is the swelling and sometimes painful gases in the stomach and intestinal tract. Serious and prolonged indiges-tion could lead to malnutrition and other complications, such as weakness, anemia, debility, and consumption.

Ginseng has a stimulant effect on the smooth muscles of the stomach and intestines; perhaps this is why ginseng has long been recognized as a *bitter tonic, stomachic,* and stimulant to the entire digestive system. In animal studies, it was found that ginseng extract caused acceleration of the gastroinestinal movement,[118,119] or increased gastric acidity.[120] The extrac-tives of ginseng leaves similarly showed a smooth muscle stimulant effect. Dr. Harding, a pioneer American ginseng user and cultivator, once said that: "Ginseng combined with the juice of a good ripe pineapple is par excellent as a treat-ment for indigestion. It stimulates the healthy secretion of pepsin, thereby insuring good digestion without incurring the habit of taking pepsin or after-dinner pills to relieve the fullness and distress so common to the American people."[121]

12
CAN GINSENG MAKE OLD PEOPLE YOUNG?

LONGEVITY

There have always been stories and legends about miraculously long lives, and about people who regained their youth. Poets in the Middle Ages wrote of a Fountain of Youth in which one could bathe and return to youth. The ancient Chinese Taoists believed that one could reach immortality by observing the doctrine of Taoism. Also the Western alchemists, the ancient inventors of chemistry (though their practice was essentially magic), pursued the dreams of eternal youth. They made it one of the three greatest goals or dreams of mankind: the magic of changing lead to gold, traveling to the moon, and discovering the elixir of life that would make old people young (rejuvenation). In the second century A.D., the Egyptian craftsmen in Alexandria were the first alchemists in history who tried desperately to convert metal into gold. Almost simultaneously and independently, the ancient Chinese Taoist monks (not pure alchemists but religious magicians) believed that gold, a miraculous medicine, was the supreme achievement on earth and they too sought to make it in a supernatural way, not for wealth but for perpetual youth and immortality. Some high priests of Toaist have spent and dedicated their whole lives searching for the "life-prolonging elixir." Unfortunately, neither the Western alchemists nor the Chinese Taoists achieved their dreams. However, as time passed and modern science

206

arrived, two of the old dreams of mankind began to come true. Even the third dream — longevity and youthfulness — is slowly coming true.

A remarkable article entitled "Every Day Is a Gift when You Are over 100" appeared in the January 1973 issue of *National Geographic Magazine*.[1] It represents the contemporary oldest people in the world, most of them well over 100 years of age. In the article, Dr. Alexander Leaf of Harvard University, found that most people living in the Caucasus of southern Russia were more than 100 years old. If we can live healthily, it has been said that the maximum life expentancy of the human species is about 140 years. In other words, you can live an extra sixty or even eighty years if you can live happily and healthily. Would you call it an extra gift from God?

Gerontologists are sometimes asked if they really think that it is a good idea to make people live longer. Perhaps the legislators have the same question. Obviously, it would raise many socioeconomic problems concerning population, welfare, and medical care. These problems would not be as un-manageable if the aged population were kept healthy. If we only make people live longer, like Tithonus, to live an isolated, unrespected, unhappy and suffering life, it certainly is not a good thing. On the other hand, if the aged people are physical-ly healthy, mentally clear, and active in their seventies and eighties, they would be very beneficial and valuable to society. They have rich experience and sound judgment, and these people can do more constructive work, carry out more respon-sibilities, and accomplish more than the young generation.

It would be wonderful to preserve a youthful body for as long as possible, but how would you reach this goal? Slowing down aging, of course, is the way to do it. You don't look young if you don't feel young. To feel young means to be healthy. Why are the native Abkhasians of the Caucasus Mountains long-lived? Because they live a way of life that is close to nature. They use all natural substances, no artificial or synthetic chemicals. Their foods, fruits, and vegetables are organically grown. They use herbal medicine, herbal tea, honey, garlic, and do not eat much meat. They also enjoy physical activity in their advanced years.

Chinese gymnastic exercise, particularly *t'ai-chi-chuan*, is said to have a therapeutic effect. The correct breathing and the mild movement during the exercise will stimulate blood circulation, thus bringing nourishment to all parts of your body so that the muscles, ligaments, joints, and organs are exercised and strengthened. Diseases such as hypertension, indigestion, tuberculosis, and ailments of the joints and muscles can be improved or cured.

The ancient Chinese lived long lives, particularly vegetarian Buddhist monks and Taoists. The following paragraph cited from the classical Chinese medical treatise, the *Huang Ti Nei Ching Su Wan, (The Yellow Emperor's Cannon of Internal Medicine)*,[2] may give you some idea how the ancient Chinese attain their longevity:

> The Yellow Emperor, Huang Ti, once addressed T'ien Shih, the divinely inspired teacher or Master of Heaven in Taoism: "I have heard that in ancient times the people lived to be over a hundred years, and yet they remained active and did not become decrepit in their activities. But nowadays, people reach only half of that age and yet become decrepit and failing. Is it because the world changes from generation to generation? Or is it that mankind is becoming negligent?" The medical minister of the emperor, Ch'i Po, answered: "In ancient times, those people who understood *Tao* [The Right Way] patterned themselves upon the Yin and the Yang, and they lived in harmony with the arts of divination. The ancient people kept their bodies united with their soul, so as to fulfill their allotted span completely, measuring unto a hundred years before they passed away. Nowadays, people are not like this; they use wine as beverage, and they adopt recklessness and unusual behavior. They enter the chamber in an intoxicated condition [overindulge]; their passions exhaust their vital forces; their cravings dissipate their true essence; they do not know how to find contentment within themselves; they are not skilled in the control of their spirit. They devote all their attention to the amusement of their minds, thus cutting themselves off from the joy of long life. Their rising [work] and retiring [rest] is without regularity. For these reasons they reach only one-half of the hundred years. . . ."

GINSENG TONIC FOR THE AGED

As people age, they tend to become physically unfit, mentally impaired, and fall prey to more diseases than the young. We can recognize aging by grey or white hair, weakened muscles, wrinkled skin, loss of hearing, loss of teeth, loss of vigor, and lessening of our power to stay well and recover completely after illness. Also, it is common that the efficiency of the individual organs and the body as a whole lessens with age. More and more organic diseases, as a result of deficiencies of the organs, deterioration of the immune systems, and degeneration of the organism, emerge with age. For instance, digestive function diminishes, enzyme induction slows, physical and mental capacities weaken, and endocrine (glandular) disorders are common in the middle-aged and the aged. The decline of gonadal function, or sexual impotency, is the most notable common hormonal disease of the aged.[3]

In the United States, people over sixty five years of age are considered aged, and people between forty five and sixty-four are considered middle-aged. There are at present about twenty million Americans who are aged, and about forty-two million Americans who are middle-aged. These sixty-two million senior citizens (constitute approximately thirty-one percent of the total population) are bound to have different physical and mental problems.[4] What are the most important factors regulating one's life when he is old? Not too long ago, the National Council on the Aging (NCOA) commissioned Louis Harris and Associates, Inc., to conduct a major national survey aimed at gaining a better understanding of aging and the reality of old age in the United States. The survey findings indicate that age seems to play a minor role affecting life satisfaction, but poor health is the most serious problem in the aged.[5]

Although ginseng does not confer eternal life, it is, in fact, an excellent remedy of tonification for the aging and the aged. The ancient Chinese doctors claimed: "Ginseng restores exhausted power, making old people young. . . ." It sounds unbelievable to you and me. However, more and more scientific research reveals the secrets of ginseng: ginseng indeed possesses the virtues above. We know, among other effects, that (1) ginseng has antistress and adaptogenic powers; (2) ginseng stimulates the synthesis of protein, bone marrow DNA, and blood cells, thus functioning as a poweful hematinic agent; (3) ginseng is a metabolic regulator for protein, carbohydrate, and fat, including cholesterol; (4) the tonic effect of ginseng keeps the organs (five viscera) and endocrine glands in a harmonious working order. These properties are absolutely essential in maintaining good health thus to make you feel young. Only recently, we also learned that ginseng contains certain unknown principles that are capable of delaying degeneration of primary human amnion (PHA) cells *in virtro*.[6] If the degeneration effect of cells is also delayed *in vivo*, then ginseng is indeed capable of making old people young, and we can no longer be skeptical about the Chinese herbal medicine as being based on superstition.

REFERENCES

CHAPTER 1

1. *Chung Yao Chih (Chinese Herbal Drugs),* Chinese Academy of Medical Sciences, Institute of Pharmacology, ed., Jen Min Wei Sheng Press, Vol. 1, Peking, 1959.

2. *Ch'ang Yung Chung Yao (Commonly Used Chinese Drugs),* Ch'eng Tu Chung I Hsueh Yuan, ed., Shanghai Jen Min Wei Sheng Press, Shanghai, 1973.

3. Bowers, John Z., *Chemtech*: August, 1974, p. 458.

4. "Herbal Pharmacology in the People's Republic of China", National Academy of Sciences, Washington, D.C., 1975, p. 12.

5. Veith, I., *J. Am. Med. Assoc., 228*: 1577 (1974).

6. Huard, P. and M. Wong, *Chinese Medicine*, McGraw-Hill Book Co., New York, 1973.

7. Veith, Ilza, *Huang Ti Nei Ching Su Wen (The Yellow Emperor's Classic of International Medicine),* (translation) University of California Press, Berkeley, 1966.

8. Smith, A. J., *Brit. Med. J., 2*: 367 (1974).

9. Claus, E. P., *et al., Pharmacognosy,* Lea and Febiger Publishers, Philadelphia, 1970.

10. Martin, E. W. and E. F. Cook (eds.), *Remington's Practice of Pharmacy,* 11th ed., The Mack Publishing Co., Easton, Pa., 1956, pp. 7-10.

11. Hsu, Kuo-chun and Chao, Shou-hsun, *Pharmacognosy,* Hong Kong Wei Sheng Press, Hong Kong, 1971, pp. 1-34.

12. Hsu, Kuo-chun, *et al., Yao Ts'ai Hsueh,* Jen Min Wei Sheng Press, Peking, 1961.

13. Croizier, R. C., *Traditional Medicine in Modern China,* Harvard University Press, Cambridge, 1968.

14. Horn, Dr. J. S., *Away With All Pests,* Monthly Review Press, New York, 1971.

15. Mao, Tze-tung, *Instruction on Public Health Work*, People's Health Press, June 3, 1967, p. 9.

16. Bowers, J. Z. and E. F. Purcell, (eds.), *Medicine and Society in China*, William F. Fell Co., Philadelphia, 1974.

17. Li, C. P., *Chinese Herbal Medicine*, U. S. Department of Health, Education, and Welfare, Publication No. (NIH) 75-732, 1974.

18. Wright, R. A., *The New York Times*, September 13, 1972.

CHAPTER 2

1. Li, Shih-chen, *Pen-ts'ao Kang-mu*, Shang-wu Press, Shanghai, China, Vol. 12 (original), 1970.

2. Wallnöfner, H. and A. von Rottauscher, *Chinese Folk Medicine*, the New American Library, Inc., New York, 1972, p. 44.

3. Brekhman, I.I., "Panax Ginseng," *Medgiz*, (Leningrad), 182, (1957).

4. Brekhman, I. I. and I. V. Dardynov, *Ann. Rev. Pharmacol.*, *9*: 419 (1969).

5. *Chung-Kuo Yao-hsueh Ta-tzu-tien (The Encyclopedia of Chinese Herb Medicine)*, Vol. I. Hong Kong I-Yao Weisheng Press, Hong Kong, 1972.

6. Grushvitzky, I. V., *J. Bot.*, USSR, *44*: 1694 (1959).

7. Wang, K. H., *Yao Hsueh T'ung Pao*, *1*: 264 (1953).

8. Li, C. P. *Amer. J. Chin. Med.*, *1:* 249 (1973).

9. *Herbal Pharmacology in the People's Republic of China*, National Academy of Sciences, Washington, D. C., 1975, p. 48.

10. Fournier, P., *La Nature* (Paris), 244 (1940).

11. Baranov, A., *Econ. Bot.*, *20*: 403 (1966).

12. Hsu, Kuo-chun and Chao, Shou-hsun, *Pharmacognosy*, Hong Kong Wei-sheng Press, Hong Kong, 1971, pp. 143-149.

13. Smith, F. P. and G. A. Stuart, *Chinese Medicinal Herbs*, Georgetown Press, San Francisco, 1973, pp 15-17.

14. Tan, Peh-yuan, "Collection of Chinese Medicine Papers on Ginseng," *Huang-han-I-hsueh ts'ung-shu*, Vol. 14, Chingyo Press, Taipei, 1970.

15. Williams, L. O., *Econ. Bot.*, *11*: 344 (1957).

16. Smith, F. P. and G. A. Stuart, *op cit.*: p. 304.

17. Imamura, T., *Ninjin Shinso*, Korean Ginseng Monopoly Bureau Press, Kae-Jo, 1923.

18. Imamura, T., *Ninjin-shi, (History of Ginseng)*, Vol. 5, "Medical and Pharmaceutical Aspects," Shibunkaku, Kyoto, 1971, pp. 232-242.

19. Smith, F. P. and G. A. Stuart, *Chinese Medicinal Herbs*, Georgetown Press, San Francisco, 1973, pp. 301-304.

20. Smith, F. P. and G. A. Stuart, *op. cit.*, p. 400.

21. Hsu, Kuo-chun and Chao, Shou-hsun, *op. cit.*, p. 463-465.

22. Smith, F. P. and G. A. Stuart, *op. cit.*, p. 392.

23. Smith, F. P. and G. A. Stuart, *op. cit.*, p. 414.

24. Smith, F. P. and G. A. Stuart, *op. cit.*, p. 341.

25. Hsu, Kuo-chun and Chao, Shou-hsun, *op. cit.*, p. 460-461.

CHAPTER 3

1. Wagner, E. W. in *The Encyclopedia Americana*, Americano Crop., New York, Vol. 16, p. 528 f.

2. Li, Shih-chen, *Pen-ts'ao Kang-mu*, Shang-wu Press, Shanghai, Vol. 12 (original), 1970.

3. Yoon, J. H. in "Korean Ginseng Science Symposium," Korean Society of Pharmacognosy, Seoul, 1974, pp. 227-239.

4. Read, B. E., *Pharm. J.*, *117*: 671, (1926).

5. "Koreanishe Ginseng", a Foreign Press article of Korean ginseng, Office of Monopoly, Seoul, 1974.

6. Imamura, T. *Nin-jin Shin-so*, Office of Monopoly, Kae-jo, Korea, 1923.

7. "Korean Ginseng," Abstract of papers of first ginseng symposium, Seoul, Korea, September 1974.

8. Kim, S. K. in "Korean Ginseng Science Symposium," Korean Society of Pharmacognosy, Seoul, 1974, pp. 207-226.

CHAPTER 4

1. Hall, J. W. in *The Encyclopedia Americana*, Americano Corp., New York, Vol. 15, pp. 814-24.

2. Imamura, T., *Nin-jin shih, (History of Ginseng)*, Vol. 5, "Medical and Pharmaceutical Aspect," Shibunkaku, Kyoto, 1971.

3. Imamura, T., *Ninijin Shin-so*, Office of Monopoly Press, Kae-jo, Korea, 1923.

4. Fuji Marketing Report, July, 1975.

5. Brekhman, I. I., *Ind. J. Publ. Health.*, *9*: 148 (1965).

6. Sandberg, F., *Planta Medica*, *24*: 392 (1974).

7. Brekhman, I. I. in "Pharmacology of Oriental Plant", K. K. Chen and B. Murkerji, eds., Pergamon Press, New York, 1965.

8. Hara, H., *Shokubutsu Kenkyu Zasshi*, 45: 197 (1970).

9. Kondo, N., J. Shoji, and O. Tanaka, *Chem. Pharm. Bull.,* 21: 2702 (1973).

10. Hsu, Kuo-chun and Chao, Shou-hsun, *Pharmacognosy,* Hong Kong Wei-sheng Press, Hong Kong, 1971, pp. 458-459.

11. Smith, F. P. and G. A. Stuart, *Chinese Medicinal Herbs,* Gerogetown Press, San Francisco, 1973, p. 201-202.

CHAPTER 5

1. Hart, B. L., in *Cyclopedia of Farm Crops,* L. H. Bailey, ed. The Macmillan Co., New York, 1922.

2. Fournier, P., *La Nature,* (Paris), p. 244 (1940).

3. Harding, A. R., *Ginseng and Other Medicinal Plants,* Emporium Pub., Boston, 1972.

4. Baugart, R. A., in *Milwaukee Journal,* December 13, 1974.

5. Schroger, A. W., "Ginseng: A Pioneer Resource," *Wisconsin Aca. Sci., Arts and Lett.,* 57: 65 (1963).

6. Garriques, S. S. *Ann Chem. Pharm., 90*: 231 (1854).

7. Vogel, V. J., *American Indian Medicine*, University of Oklahoma Press, Norman, 1970, pp. 307-10.

8. Stockberger, W. W., "Ginseng Culture," *Farmers Bulletin No. 1184,* U. S. Department of Agriculture, Washington, D. C., U. S. Government Publishing Office, 1921, revised 1949.

9. Williams, L., "Growing Ginseng," *Farmers Bulletin No. 2201,* U. S. Department of Agriculture, U. S. Government Printing Office, 1964, revised 1973.

CHAPTER 6

1. Savag, W. N., *Penn. Angular,* November, 1969, pp. 18-22.

2. Time Special Bicentennial Issue: September 26, 1976, p. 44.

3. Camplin, P., "Ginseng Hunting: A Lost Art," in *Our Heritage,* Kentucky October, 1965.

4. Schorger, A. W., "Ginseng: A Pioneer Resource," *Wis. Acad. Sci. Arts and Lett.,* 57: 65 (1969).

5. Nash, G. V., "American Ginseng: Its Commercial History, Protection and Cultivation," U. S. Department of Agriculture, Div. Botany, *Bulle-*

tin No. *16*, Revised edition, U. S. Government Printing Office, Washington, D. C.

6. Lass, W. E., "Ginseng Rush in Minnesota," *Minn. Hist., 41:* 249 (1969).

7. Harding, A. R., *Ginseng and Other Medicinal Plants,* Emporium Publications, Boston, 1972, pp. 121-132.

8. Stockberger, W. W., "Ginseng Culture," U. S. Department of Agriculture, *Bulletin No. 1184,* U. S. Government Printing Office, 1921, revised, 1949.

9. Williams, L. O., "Ginseng," *Econ. Bot., 11:* 344 (1957).

10. U. S. Department of Commerce, extract from U. S. Exports, *Schedule B., Commodity by Country, EQ 629, 2928010,* "Ginseng," January to December, U. S. Government Printing Office, Washington, D.C.

11. *Agriculture Situation,* S.R.S. U. S. Department of Agriculture, Washington, D. C., May 1975, p. 12.

12. Aston, *Pharm. J., 15:* 732 (1885).

13. Jones, B., "Ginseng: Seoul's Oldest Export," *New York Times,* March 14, 1971.

14. *Statistical Year Book of Foreign Trade,* Department of Customs Administration, Republic of Korea, 1974.

15. *Fuji Marketing Report,* July, 1975.

16. *Import Alert,* FDA Headquarters, Field Compliance Branch January 28, 1975.

CHAPTER 7

1. Hong, S. K. in "Korean Ginseng Science Symposium," Korean Society of Pharmacognosy, Seoul, 1974, pp. 37-54.

2. Stockberger, W. W. in "Ginseng Culture," *Farmer's Bulletin No. 1184,* U. S. Department of Agriculture, 1921, Revised 1941.

3. Williams, L. in "Growing Ginseng," *Farmer's Bulletin No. 2201,* U. S. Department of Agriculture, 1964, Revised 1973, U. S. Government Printing Office, Washington, D.C.

4. Harding, A. R.: "Ginseng and Other Medicinal Plants," Emporium Publications, Boston, 1972.

5. King, W., "Georgean Farm," *The New York Times,* October 11, 1975.

6. Baranov, A., *Econ. Bot., 20:* 403 (1966).

7. (a) Bukovac and Wittwer, Quarterly Bulletin Michigan Agricultural Experiment Station, *39:* 307 (1956).
   (b) Merritt, *J. Ag. Food Chem., 6:* 184 (1958).

8. Grushvitskii, I. V. and R. S. Limar, *J. Bot.,* USSR, *50:* 215 (1965).

9. Osumi, T. and Y. Miwazawa, *Nogyo Oyobi Engei*, *35*: 723, (1960) via *Chem. Abstr.*, *56*: 2731g (1962).

10. Nikolaeva, M. G., I. V. Grushvitskii and V. M. Bogdanova, *Bot. Zh.* (Leningrad), *57*: 1082 (1972) via *Chem. Abstr. 78*: 25215x (1973).

11. Kuribayashi, T., M. Okamura and H. Ohashi, *Shoyakugaku Zasshi, 25*: 87-94 (1971).

12. Kuribayashi, T. and H. Ohashi, *ibid.*: 95 (1971).

13. Kuribayashi, T. and M. Okamura and H. Ohashi, *ibid*: 102 (1971).

14. Kuribayashi, T. and H. Ohashi, *ibid*: 110 (1971).

CHAPTER 8

1. Jones, B., *The New York Times*, March 14, 1971.

2. *The New York Times*, April 25, 1972.

3. King. W., *The New York Times*, October 11, 1975.

4. Geczl, M. L., *The Wall Street Journal*, September 9, 1975.

5. *Milwaukee Journal*, April 8, 1973.

6. Baumgart, R. A., *Milwaukee Journal*, December 13, 1974.

7. Gathercoal, E. N., and E. H. Wirth, *Pharmacognosy*, Lea and Febiger, Philadelphia, 1936.

8. Youngken, H. W., *Texbook of Pharmacognosy*, The Blakiston Company, Philadelphia, 1950, pp. 607-609.

9. Claus, E. P., U. E. Tyler, and L. R. Brady, *Pharmacognosy*, Lea and Febiger, Philadelphia, 1970, pp. 113-114.

10. *United States Pharmacopeia*, Mack Publishing Company, Easton, Pennsylvania.

11. *United States Dispensatory*, Mack Publishing Company, Easton, Pennsylvania.

12. *National Formulary*, J. P. Lippincott Company, Philadelphia.

13. *Index Medicus*, U. S. Government Printing Office, Washington, D. C., 20402.

14. *Chemical Abstract*, Chemical Abstract Service, Columbus, Ohio.

15. Webb, R. G. to J. P. Hou, Correspondence, April 18, 1975.

16. Duke, J. A. to J. P. Hou, Correspondence, June 2, 1975.

17. Garriques, S., *Ann. Chem. Pham.*, *90*: 231 (1854).

18. Jackson, J. R., *The Pharm. J.*, 86 (1875).

19. Brekhman, I. I., *Ind. J. Pub. Health*, *9*: 148 (1965).

20. "Proceedings of International Ginseng Symposium," The Central Research Institute, Office of Monopoly, Seoul, Korea, 1974.

References 217

21. "Scientific Documentation of Panax Ginseng C. A. M.", Pharmaton, Ltd., Lugano-Bioggio, Switzerland, 1975.

CHAPTER 9

1. Rafinesque, *Am. J. Pharm.*, *26*: 510 (1854).
2. Garriques, S. S., *ibid.*, 511 (1854), *Ann. Chem. Pharm.*, *90*: 231 (1854).
3. Davydow, *Pharm. Zeitscher. Russland*, *29*: 97 (1889).
4. Inoue, M., *J. Pharm. Soc., Japan*, *242*: 326 (1902).
5. Fujitani, K., *J. Tokyo Med. Assoc.*, *2*: 43 (1905).
6. Asahina, U. and B. Taguchi, *J. Pharm. Soc., Japan*, *25*: 547 (1906).
7. Kondo, H. and G. Tanaka, *ibid.*, *35*: 779 (1915).
8. Kondo, H. and S. Yamaguchi, *ibid.*, *38*: 747 (1918).
9. Kondo, H. and U. Amano, *ibid.*, *40*: 1027 (1920).
10. Abe, K. and I. Saito, *Japan Med. World*, *2*: 166 (1922).
11. Yonekawa, M., *ibid*, *785* (1926).
12. Kotake, M., *J. Chem. Soc., Japan*, *51*: 357 (1930); *51*: 396 (1930).
13. Sakai, W., *Tokyo Igakukai Zasshi*, *31*: 1 (1917).
14. Sakai, W., *Japan Med. Lit.*, *3*: 27 (1918).
15. Sakai, W., *Ijishimpun*, *990*: 112 (1918).
16. Sakai, W., *Japan Med. Lit.*, *5*: 6 (1920).
17. Shibata, S., *Tampakushitsu*, *12*: 32 (1967).
18, Tanaka, O., *Taisha*, *10*: 548 (1973).
19. Han, B. H., in "Korean Ginseng Symposium,; Korean Society of Pharmacognosy, 1974, pp. 81-111.
20. Claus, E. P., V. E. Tayler, and L. R. Brady, *Pharmacognosy*, Lea and Feibiger Company, Philadelphia, 6th ed., Chapter 4, (1970).
21. Trease, G. E. and W. C. Evans, *Pharmacognosy*, The Williams and Wilkins Company, Baltimore, Chapter 12, (1972).
22. Brekhman, I. I., "Panax Ginseng," *Medgiz*, (Leningrad): 182 (1957).
23. Naidenova, I. N., V. A. Andreeva, V. T. Bykov, S. P. Versen, E. S. Zyakhov, and V. F. Chernil, *Izvest. Acad. Nauk,* USSR, Otdel Khim Nauk: 1403 (1957).
24. Elyakov, G. B., L. I. Strigina, A. J. Khorlin and N. K. Kochetkov, *Izvest. Acad. Nauk*, S.S.S.R., Ser. Khim Nauk: 1125, 2054 (1962).
25. Elyakov, G. B., L. I. Strigina, N. I. Uvarova, V. E. Vskovsky, A. K.

Dzizenko, and N. K. Koochetkov, *Tetrahedron Lett.*, No. 48: 3591 (1964).

26. Elyakov, G. B., A. K. Dzizenko, and Yu, N. Elkin, *ibid.*, No. 1: 141 (1966).

27. Andreev, L. V., L. I. Slepyan and I. K. Nikitina, *Rast. Resur.*, 10: 126 (1974).

28. Fujita, M., H. Itokawa, and S. Shibata, *J. Pharm. Soc., Japan 82*: 1634, 1638 (1962).

29. Shibata, S., M. Fujita, H. Itokawa, O. Tanaka, and T. Ishii, *Tetrahedron Lett.*, No. 10: 419 (1962).

30. Shibata, S., O. Tanaka, M. Nagai, and T. Ishii, *ibid.*, No. 26: 1239 (1962).

31. Shibata, S., O. Tanaka, M. Nagai, and T. Ishii, *Chem. Pharm. Bull.*, 11: 762 (1963).

32. Shibata, S., M. Fujita, H. Itokawa, O. Tanaka, and T. Ishii, *ibid.*, 11: 759 (1963).

33. Shibata, S., O. Tanaka, M. Sado, and S. Tsushima, *Tetrahedron Lett.*, No. 12: 795 (1963).

34. Tanaka, B., M. Nagai, and S. Shibata, *ibid.*, No. 33: 2291 (1964).

35. Shibata, S., O. Tanaka, K. Some, Y. Iida, T. Ando, and H. Nakamura, *ibid.*, No. 3, 207 (1965).

36. Sanada, S., *et al., Chem. Pharm. Bull*, 22: 421, 2407 (1974).

37. Shibata, S., *et al., Chem. Pharm. Bull.*, 14: 595 (1966).

38. Iida, Y., O. Tanaka, and S. Shibata, *Tetrahedron Lett.*, No. 52: 5449 (1968).

39. Wagner-Jauregg, T., and M. Roth, *Pharm. Acta. Helv.*, 38: 125 (1963).

40. Lin, Y. T., *J. Chin. Chem. Soc.*, (Taiwan), 8: 109 (1961).

41. Horhammer, L., H. Wagner, and B. Lay, *Pharm. Ztg.*, 106: 1307 (1961).

42. Takahashi, M., K. Isoi, M. Yoshikura and T. Osugi, *J. Pharm. Soc., Japan, 81*: 771 (1961).

43. Takahashi, M., *et al., ibid.*, 84: 752, 757 (1964).

44. Takahashi, M., and M. Yoshikura, *ibid.*, 86: 1051, 1053 (1966).

45. Euler, H. and E. Nordenson, *Z. Physiol. Chem.*, 56: 223 (1908).

46. Ahn, Y. P. and C. C. Chung, *Kor. J. Chem. Soc.*, 14: 281 (1970).

47. Takiura, K. and I. Nakagawa, *J. Pharm. Soc., Japan, 83*: 298 (1963).

48. *Ibid.*, 83: 301 (1963).

49. *Ibid.*, 83: 305, 308 (1963).

50. Ovodov, Yu. S. and T. F. Solov'eva, *Khim. Prir. Soedin.* 2: 299 (1966).

51. Solov'eva, T. F., L. V. Arsenyuk, Yu. S. Ovodov. *Carbohyd. Res. 10:* 13 (1969).

52. Solov'eva, T., *et al. Khim. Prir. Soedin.*, *5:* 201 (1969).

53. Park, M. S. *In-Sam-Mun-Hun-Teuk-Zip,* Central Technical Research Institute, the Office of Monopoly, Seoul, p. 1, (1969).

54. Lee, C. Y. and T. Y. Lee, *Sym. Photochem. Proc. Meeting,* University of Hong Kong, p. 171 (1961).

55. Gstirner, F. and H. J. Vogt, *Arch. Pharm.* (Weinheim), *300:* 371 (1967).

56. Gstirner, F., and W. Brown, *ibid.,* *296:* 384 (1963).

57. Wong, Y. C., *J. Am. Pharm. Assoc.,* *10:* 431 (1921).

58. Takatori, K., *et al.,* *Chem. Pharm. Bull.,* *11:* 1342 (1963).

59. Gstirner, F. and H. J. Vogt, *Arch. Pharm.* (Weinham), *299:* 936 (1966).

60. White, Abraham, P. Handler, E. I. Smith, *Principles of Biochemistry,* Fourth Ed., McGraw-Hill Book Co., New York, 1968, p. 540.

61. Goto, M., *J. Pharm. Soc., Japan, 77:* 467, 471, (1957).

62. Kim, Y. E., S. K. Juhn, and B. J. An, *Yakhak Hoeji (J. Pharm. Soc., Korea), 8:* 80 (1964).

63. Kim, Y. E., and M. O. Her, *ibid., 8:* 85 (1964).

64. Nomura, S. and Y. Oshima, *J. Chosen Med. Assoc., 20:* No. 3 (1930).

65. Jhang, J. J., E. J. Staba, and J. Y. Kim, *In Vitro, 9:* 253 (1974).

66. Pijck, J. and J. I. Kim, *J. Pharm. Belg., 19:* 3 (1964).

67. Pijck, J., and A. Claeys, Mededel. Landbouwhogeschool Opzoekingssta. Staat. Gent. *30:* 1295 (1965).

68. Yamaguchi, I., *J. Chosen Med. Assoc.,* No. 85, 125, 568 (1928).

69. Yoshizaki, M., *et al., Shoyakugaku Zasshi, 27:* 110 (1973).

70. Namba, T., *et al., J. Pharm. Soc., Japan, 94:* 252 (1974).

71. Komatsu, M. and T. Tomimori, *Shoyakugaku Zasshi, 20:* 21 (1966).

72. Komatsu, M. and Y. Makiguchi, *J. Pharm. Soc., Japan, 89:* 122 (1969).

73. Nomura S. and Y. Oshima, *J. Chosen Med. Assoc., 21:* 558 (1931).

74. *Ibid.,* 553, (1931).

75. Min, P. A., *Folia Pharmacol, Japan, 11:* 238, 256 (1931).

76. Shibata, S., *et al., J. Pharm. Soc., Japan, 85:* 753 (1965).

77. Kin, K., *J. Chosen Med. Assoc., 21:* No. 5, (1931), via *Ninjinshi* Vol *5:* p. 602.

78. Torney, H. J. and F. M. Y. Cheng, *St. Bonaventure Sci. Studies, 7:* 9 (1939).

79. Kim, J. Y. and E. J. Staba in Proceedings of International Ginseng Symposium - 1974, The Central Research Institute, Office of Monopoly, Republic of Korea, pp. 77-93.

80. Kim, Jung-Yun, "Saponin and Sapogenin Distribution in American Ginseng Plant," Ph. D. thesis - 1974, The University of Minnesota, Xerox University Microfilm, Ann Arbor, 1975.

81. Murayama, Y. and T. Itagaki, *J. Pharm. Soc., Japan 43:* 783 (1923).

82. Murayama, Y. and S. Tanaka, *J. Pharm. Soc., Japan, 47:* 526 (1927).

83. Aoyama, S., *ibid., 50:* 1065 (1930).

84. Kotake, M., *ibid., 50:* 396 (1930).

85. Kitasota, I., and S. C. Sone, *Acta Phytochim., Japan, 6:* 179 (1932).

86. Kuwata, S. and Matsukawa, *J. Pharm. Soc., Japan, 54:* 211 (1934).

87. Kondo, N., *et al., Chem. Pharm. Bull., 18:* 1558 (1970), *19:* 1103 (1971).

88. Kochetkov, N. K., A. J. Khorlin and V. E. Vaskovsky, *Tetrahedron Lett., 713* (1962).

89. Kondo, N., J. Shoji, and O. Tanaka, *Chem. Pharm. Bull., 21:* 2702 (1973).

90. Brekhman, I. I. and I. V. Dardymov, *Lloyda, 32:* 46 (1969).

91. Brekhman, I. I., "Eleutherococcus," The Nauka Publishing House, Leningrad, (1968).

92. Ovodov, Yu. S., *et al., Khim. Prirodnih Soedin, 1:* 63 (1967).

CHAPTER 10

1. Wang, P. H., *Acta. Pharm. Sinica, 12:* 477, (1965).

2. Brekhman, I. I., *Medgiz,* Leningrad: 182, (1957).

3. Brekhman, I. I., *Med. Sci. Serv., 4:* 17, (1967).

4. Brekhman, I. I., and I. V. Dardymov, *Lloyda, 32:* 46, (1969).

5. Brekhman, I. I., and I. V. Dardymov, *Ann. Rev. Pharmacol., 9:* 419, (1969).

6. Lazarev, N. V., *7th All-Union Congr. of Physiol. Biochem. Pharmacol., Medgiz,* Moscow: 579 pp., 1947.

7. Yonekawa, M., *Keijo J. Med., 6:* 785 (1926).

8. Kitagawa, H. and R. Iwaki, *Nippon Yakurigaku Zasshi,* (Folia Pharmacol., Japan), *59:* 348, 1963.

9. Hong, S. A. and H. Y. Cho in "Korean Ginseng Science Symposium", Korean Society of Pharmacognosy, Seoul, 1974, pp. 113-139.

10. Kaku, T., *et al., Arzneim-Forsch., 25:* 539, (1975).

11. *Industry Week,* January 30, 1975.

12. Leff, D. N., *Med. World News, 16:* 74, March 24, 1975.

13. *Med. World News, 16:* 103, February 24, 1975.

14. Cobb, S. and R. M. Rose, *J. Am. Med. Assoc., 224:* 489, (1973).

15. Sung, C. Y. and H. C. Chi, *Acta Physiol Sinica, 22:* 155 (1958).

16. Liu, K. T. and C. Y. Sung, *Ibid., 25:* 129 (1962).

17. Chang, T. H. and T. H. Kao, *J. Chin. Med. Assoc. 44:* 1040 (1958).

18. Tsung, J.Y., C. Cheng and S. Tang. *Acta Physiol. Sinica, 27:* 324 (1964).

19. Petkov, W. and D. Staneva-Stoicheva, *Proc. 2nd. Intern. pharmacol. meet.* Prague, August 20-23, 1963 Pergamion Press, N.Y., 1965, pp. 39-45.

20. Wang, P. H., *Acta Pharm. Sinica, 12:* 477 (1965).

21. Kim, B. I., *Choongang Uihak (Korean Med. J.), 8:* 107 (1963).

22. Kim, C., *Katorik Taehak Uihakpu,* Nonumnjip, *8:* 251 (1964).

23. Kim, C. C., *Katorik Taehak Uihakpu, Non mumjit, 9:* 29 (1965).

24. Yoon, H. S., and C. Kim, *ibid., 21:* 25, (1971).

25. Hu, C. Y. and C. Kim, *ibid., 12:* 49 (1967).

26. Kim, C. C., J. K. Kim, and C. Y. Hu., *ibid., 10:* 455 (1966).

27. Hu, C. Y., C. C. Kim, and J. K. Kim, *Choosin Uihak, 10:* 73 (1967).

28. Kim, C. C., J. K. Kim, and C. Y. Hu, *ibid., 10:* 57 (1967).

29. Kim, C., C. C. Kim, M. S. Kim, C. Y. Hu, and J. S. Rhe, *Lloydia, 33:* 43 (1970).

30. Kim, H. R. and W. B. Kim, *Choesin Uihak 15:* 87 (1972).

31. Kim, W. B. and H. Y. Chung, *ibid., 15:* 83 (1972).

32. Amirov, R. V. and E. B. Abdulova, *Uchenye zapskii Azerbaidzhanskogo Zast. Usoversh Urachei, 1:* 3 (1966).

33. Kim, Chung-chin *et al.. ch'oesin Uihak, 10:* 57 (1967)

34. Oshima, Yoshio, *J. Chosen Med. Assoc., 19:* 539 (1929).

35. Golikov, P. P., *Information for a Study of Ginseng and Other Drugs of the Soviet Far East, 7:* 17 (1966).

36. Hong, S. A., *Ch'oesin Uihak, 15:* 87 (1972).

37. Kim, Chung-Chin and Hyo-Koon Roh, *Katorik Taehak, Uihakpu.* Nonmunjip, *8:* 265 (1964).

38. Kim, C. C., *Korean Med. J., 11:* 51 (1966).

39. Choi, Y. C., *Seoul Uidae Chapchi, 13:* 1 (1972).

40. Chang, Pao-heng, *Yao Hsueh Hsueh Pao* (Acta Pharm. Sinica), *13:* 106 (1966).

41. Brekhaman, I. I. and N. K. Fruentov, *Farmakol. i Toksikol., 19:* suppl. 37 (1956).

42. Zhou, J. H., F. Y. Fu, and H. P. Lei, "Proceedings of the Second Inter-

national Pharmacological Meeting" in *Pharmacology of Oriental Plant,* Vol 7, K. K. Chen and B. Mukerji, eds., Pergamon Press, New York, 1965, p. 17.

43. Pichurina, R. A., *Dissertacija, Tomskiy Medicinskiy. Institut.,* Tomsk, 1963, pp. 106.

44. Brekhman, I. I. and O. I. Kirillov, *Rast. Resursy., 4:* 1 (1968).

CHAPTER 11

1. Brekhmam, I. I. and I. V. Dardymov, *Ann. Rev. Pharmacol., 9:* 419 (1969).

2. Brekhman, I. I., *Medgiz* (Leningrad), 182 (1957).

3. Brekhman, I. I. and I. V. Dardymov, *Lloyda, 32:* 46 (1969).

4. Brekhman, I. I., Material for the Study of *Panax ginseng* and Other Medicinal Plants for the Far East, *Primorskoe. Knizhnoe Izdatelstvo,* Vladivostok, *5:* 219 (1963).

5. Kitagawa, H. and R. Iwak, *Fol. Pharmacol. Jap., 59:* 348 (1963).

6. Brekhman, I. I., *Med. Sci. Serv., 4:* 17 (1967).

7. Brekhman, I. I., M. A. Grinevich and G. I. Glazunov, *Soobshch, Dalnevost, Filiala Akad.* Nauk, SSSR, Vladivostok, *19:* 135 (1963).

8. Brekhman, I. I., I. V. Dardymov, and Yu I. Dobrjakov, *Farmakol. i Toksikol., 29:* 167 (1966).

9. Sterner, W. and A. M. Kirchdorfer, *Z. Gerontol., 3:* 307, (1970).

10. Rueckert, K. H., in "Proceedings of International Ginseng Symposium," September, 1974, Seoul, The Office of Monopoly, Seoul, pp. 59-64.

11. Rueckert, K. H. in "Proceedings of International Symposium of Gerontology," April 9-12, 1975, Lugano, Switzerland.

12. Takagi, K., H. Saito, and H. Nabata, *Japan J. Pharmacol., 22:* 245 (1972).

13. Saito, H., Y. Yoshida, and K. Takagi, *ibid, 24:* 119 (1974).

14. Slepmyan, L. I., *Tr. Leningrad. Khim. Farm. Inst., 26:* 236 (1968).

15. Ed. *Brit. Med. J., 4:* 251 (1971).

16. Sharman, I. M. *et al., Br. J. Nutr., 26:* 265 (1971).

17. Lawrence, J. D., *et al., Am. J. Clin. Nutr., 28:* 205 (1975).

18. *The Med. Lett., 17:* 69, August, 1975.

19. Brekhman, I. I., *Ind. J. Publ. Health. 9:* 148 (1965).

20. Tsung, J. Y., Cheng, and Tang, Sui, *Sheng Li Hsueh Pao, 27:* 324 (1964).

21. Scicenkov, M. V., Papers on the Study of Ginseng and Other Medicinal Plants of the Far East, Vladivostok, Issue 5: p. 241, 1963.

22. "Cancer Cause and Prevention," U.S. Dept. Health, Education and Welfare, Public Health Service, Washington, D.C., 1966, p. 1.

23. "1973 Cancer Facts and Figures", New York American Cancer Society, Inc., 1973, p. 7.

24. *J. Am. Med. Assoc.*, *227:* 9, March 4, 1974.

25. Doll, R., C. Muir, and J. Waterhouse, *Cancer Incidence in Five Continents*, U.I.C.C., Geneva, 1970, or *Lancet*, January 17, 1976, p. 131.

26. Rauscher. F. J. *J. Am. Med. Assoc.*, *232:* 647 (1975).

27. *The Brit. Med. J.*, *3:* 329 (1974).

28. Leff, D. N. *Med. World News*, *16:* 74, (1975).

29. Moertel, C. G., *J. Am. Med. Assoc.*, *228:* 1290 (1974).

30. Lazarev, N. V., *Vopr. Onkol.*, *11:* 48 (1965).

31. Stukov, A. N., *ibid.*, 13: 94 (1967).

32. Mironova, A. I., *ibid.*, *9:* 42 (1963).

33. Jaremenko, K. V., *Mater,* Izuch Ahen'shonya Drugikh Lek. Sredsto Dal'nego Vostoka, No. 7: 109 (1966).

34. Maljugina, L. L., *Vopr. Onkol.*, *12:* 53 (1966).

35. Stukov, A. N., *ibid.*, *12:* 124 (1966).

36. Lee, K. D. and R. P. Huemer, *Jap. J. Pharmacol.*, *21:* 299 (1971).

37. Kent. S., *Geriatrics, 30:* 140, January, 1975.

38. *Ibid., 30:* 164, April 1975.

39. *Ibid., 30:* 155, September 1975.

40. Kolodny, R. C., *et al.*, *Diabetes, 23:* 306 (1974).

41. Brody, J. E., *The New York Times*, September 16, 1975.

42. Pfeiffer, E., *Geriatrics, 28:* 172, November, 1973.

43. Pfeiffer, E. and G. C. Davis, *J. Am. Geriatr. Soc.*, *20:* 151 (1972).

44. Pfeiffer, E., *J. Am. Geriatr. Soc.*, *22:* 481 (1974).

45. Kent, S., *Geriatrics, 30:* 96, December 1975.

46. Rhodes, P., *Brit. Med. J.*, *3:* 93, July 1975.

47. Bowers, M. B., Jr. and M. H. Van Woert, *Med. Aspects Hum. Sexual.:* 94, July, (1972).

48. Lawrence, D. M. and G. I. M. Swyer, *Brit. Med. J.*, *1:* 349, March (1974).

49. Eiberhof, *J. Pharm.*, Japan, *39:* 469 (1905).

50. Abe, K. and I. Saito, *Japan Med. World, 2:* 263 (1922).

51. Min. P. K., *Folia Pharmacol.*, Japan, *11:* 238, 256 (1931).

52. Kin, K. *J. Chosen, Med. Assoc.*, *21*, Vol. 5, 1931; *Keijo. J. Med.*, *2:* 345 (1931).

53. Imamura, Tomo, *Ninjmshih (History of Ginseng)*, Kyoto Shibunkaku, *5:* pp. 624-634 (1971).

54. Weber, U., *Suddent Apoth-Ztg.*, *78:* 645, 657, and 667 (1938).

55. Kit, S. M., *Farmkol i Toksikol.*, *25:* 629 (1962).

56. Wang, P. H., *Acta Pharm. Sinica*, *12:* 477 (1965).

57. Shibata, K., S. Tadokoro, Y. Kurihara, H. Ogawa and K. Miyashita, *Kitakanto Med. J.* (Japan), *14:* 243 (1964).

58. Yamada, M., *Japan J. Pharmacol.* *4:* 390 (1955).

59. Anguelakova, D. M., D. P. Rovesti, and D. E. Colômbo, *Aromi, Saponi, Cosmet. Aerosol.*, *53:* 275 (1971).

60. Suh, C. M., B. H. Kim, and I. S. Chang, *Taehan Saengri Hakhoe Chi.*, *7:* 37 (1973).

61. Yamamoto, M., *Taisha*, *10:* 581 (1973).

62. Kang, J. W., *Choesin Uihak*, *13:* 43 (1970).

63. Fujitani, K., *Tokyo Igakukai Zasshi*, *2:* No. 3, 43 (1905).

64. Sakai, W., *Tokyo Igaku Dai Zasshi*, *31:* 1 (1917).

65. Sakai, W., *Iji Shimbun*, *990:* 112 (1918).

66. Sakai, W., *Japan Med. Cit.*, *3:* 27 (1918) and *5:* 6 (1920).

67. Yonekawa, M., *Keijo J. Med.*, *6:* 633 and 785 (1926).

68. Sim, S. J. and J. S. Oh, *Taehan Yakrihak Chapchi*, *9:* 9 (1973).

69. Hong, S. A., *et al.*, *ibid.*, *10:* 73 (1974).

70. Lee, S. W. *ibid.*, 85 (1974).

71. Nabata, H., H. Saito, and K, Takagi, *Japan J. Pharmacol.*, *23:* 29 (1973).

72. Takagi, K., H. Saito, and M. Tsuchiya, *ibid* *22:* 339 (1972).

73. Kaku, T. *et al.*, *Arzneim. Forsch.*, *25:* 539 (1975).

74. Chu, S. K., *Yao Hsueh T'ung Pao*, *1:* 375 (1953).

75. Sandberg, F. in "Proceedings of International Ginseng Symposium", September, 1974, Seoul, The Office of Monopoly, Korea, pp. 65-67.

76. Watanabe, S., *Japan Med. Lit.*, *6:* 1 (1921).

77. Raymond-Hamet, C. R., *Acad. Sci.*, *23:* 3269 (1962).

78. Zyryanova, T. M., *Stimulyatory Tsent. Nerv. Sist.*, Tomask: 37 (1966). via Chem. Abstr. *66:* 114460 (1967).

79. Zhou, J. H., F. Y. Fu, and H. P. Lei, "Proceedings of the Second International Pharmacological Meeting," in *Pharmacology of Oriental*

Plant, vol. 7, K. K. Chen and B. Mukerji, ed. Pergamon Press. N.Y., 1965, p. 17.

80. Li, C. P. in "Chinese Herbal Medicine", U.S. Department of Health, Education and Welfare, DHEW Publication No. (NIH) 75-732, Washington, D.C., 1974, p. 36.

81. Stamler, J. in *The Encyclopedia Americana,* Americano Corp., N.Y., p. 611.

82. Karzel, K. in "Proceedings of International Ginseng Symposium" Seoul, September, 1974, The Office of Monopoly, Korea, pp. 49-55.

83. Popov, I. M. in "Proceedings of Symposium of Gerontology", Lugano, April, 1975, Pharmaton, Ltd., Lugano.

84. Metropolitan Life Insurance Statistical Bulletin, August, 1975.

85. *The New York Times,* July 4, 1975.

86. Arima, J. and S. Miyazaki, *J. Med. World, 2:* 275 (1922).

87. Kin, K., *J. Chosen. Med. Assoc., 22:* 221 (1932).

88. Wang, C. K. and H. P. Lei, *Chinese J. Int. Med., 5:* 861 (1957).

89. Wang, C. K. and H. P. Lei, Abstr. The First Congress of Society of the Chinese Physiological Sciences, 1956, pp. 37-8.

90. Sung, C. Y. and T. H. Chen, *ibid:* pp. 35.

91. Tsuao, C. and C. C. Yen, *ibid:* pp. 35-37.

92. Tsuao, C., C. C. Yen, and H. P. Lei, *Acta Pharma. Sinica, 7:* 208 (1959).

93. Liu, K. T., H. C. Chi, and C. Y. Sung, *ibid:* 213 (1959).

94. Bezdetko, G. N., T. M. Smolina, and L. D. Shuljateva, 11-12 Izdatl-stvo Tomskogo Universiteta, Tomsk, 1961.

95. Brekhman, I. I. and T. P. Oleinikova, via *Chem. Abstr., 60:* 163896b (1964).

96. Petkov, W., *Arch. Exptl. Pathol. Pharmakol., 236:* 289 (1959).

97. Petkov, W., *Arzneimittel-Forsch., 9:* 305 (1959).

98. Lee, M. S. *Korean Choong Ang. Med. J., 2:* 520 (1962).

99. Oura, H. and S. Hiai, *Taisha, 10:* 564 (1973).

100. Yokozawa, T., H. Seno, and H. Oura, *Chem. Pharm. Bull., 23:* 3095 (1975).

101. Oura, H. and S. Hiai, Proceedings of International Ginseng Symposium, Seoul, Korea, September 1974, The Office of Monopoly, Seoul, Korea pp. 23.

102. Yokozawa, T. and H. Oura, *Chem. Pharm. Bull., 24:* 987 (1976).

103. Saito, I., *Japan Med. World, 1:* 699, 1921; and ibid., *2:* 149 (1922).

104. Abe, K. and I. Saito, ibid., *2:* 263 (1922).

105. Shass, E. Yu., *Feldsh i Akush, 11:* 1952.

106. Unpublished Clinical Research Reports on Ginseng from Yamanouchi Pharmaceutical Co. Tokyo, Japan, 1975.

107. Bentler, E. in *The Encyclopedia Americana,* Americano Corp., N.Y., Vol. 1, p. 831.

108. Harant, Z. and J. V. Goldberger, *J. Am. Geriatr. Soc., 23:* 127 (1975).

109. Kin, K., *J. Chosen Med. Assoc., 21:* 647, 873, and 1131 (1931).

110. Kim, H. r., *Ch'oesin Uihak, 15:* 70 (1972).

111. Brekhman, I. I., *Proc. 2nd. Int. Pharmacol. Meet.,* Prague, August 20-23, 1963, Pergamon Press, 1965, pp. 97-102.

112. Ohasi, K. and H. Oura, *Japanese Patent,* 7031, 314, October 9, 1970.

113. Oura, H., and S. Nakashima, *Chem. Pharm. Bull., 20:* 980 (1972).

114. Oura, H., S. Hiai and H. Seno, *ibid., 19:* 1598 (1971).

115. Oura, H., *Japan J. Clinical Med., 25:* 2849 (1967).

116. Shida, K., *Clin. Endocr., 18:* 773 (1970).

117. Arich, S., *Taisha, 10:* 596 (1973).

118. Kitagawa, H. and R. Iwaki, *J. Yakurigaku Zasshi (Japan J. Pharmacol.), 59:* 348 (1963).

119. Petkov, W., *Arzneim-Forsch, 11:* 288 and 418 (1961).

120. Ko, Y. W., *Korean J. Intern. Med., 12:* 187 (1969).

121. Harding, A. R. in *Ginseng and Other Medicinal Plants,* Emporium Pub., Boston, 1972, p. 167.

CHAPTER 12

1. Leaf, A., *National Geographic Magazine,* January 1973, p. 93.

2. Veith, I., in *The Yellow Emperor's Classic of International Medicine,* a translation of *Hung Ti Nei Ching Su Wen,* University of California Press, Berkley, 1973, pp. 97-99.

3. Green, M. F., *Brit. Med. J., 1:* 232 (1974).

4. Botwinick, J., *Geriatrics, 29:* 124 (1974).

5. Beverley, E. V., *Geriatrics, 30:* 116 (1975).

6. Yuan, G. C. and R. S. Chang, *J. Gerontol., 24:* 82 (1969).

GLOSSARY

ACUPUNCTURE: The ancient practice, especially as carried on by the Chinese, of piercing parts of the body with needles in seeking to treat disease or relieve pain.

ADAPTOGEN: A substance causing a state of nonspecific increased resistance (SNIR) of the organism to adverse stresses of various origin.

ADENOMA: A benign tumor of glandular origin.

ADRENALECTOMY: Surgical removal of an adrenal gland.

AGLYCONE: The nonsugar portion of a glycoside.

ALKALOIDS: Nitrogenous crystalline or oily compounds, usually basic in character, such as atropine, morphine, quinine, etc.

ALTERNATIVE (as a drug): Gradually changing, or tending to change, a morbid state of the functions to a healthy person.

AMNION CELLS: Cells composing the thin, translucent wall of the fluid-filled sac for the protection of the embryo.

ANALOG: Part having the same function as another but differing in structure and origin.

ANDROGEN: A male sex hormone or synthetic substance that can give rise to masculine characteristics.

ANEMIA: A condition in which there is a reduction of the number of red blood corpuscles or of the total amount of hemoglobin in the bloodstream or both, resulting in a paleness, generalized weakness, etc.

ANTAGONISM: A mutually opposing action that can take place between organisms, muscles, drugs, etc.

ANTAGONISTIC: Showing antagonism; acting in opposition.

ANXIETY: A state of being uneasy, apprehensive, or worried about what may happen; in psychiatry, an intense state of this kind,

227

characterized by varying degrees of emotional disturbance and psychic tension.

APHRODISIAC: Any drug or other agent arousing or increasing sexual desire.

APOPLEXY: Sudden paralysis with total or partial loss of consciousness and sensation, caused by the breaking or obstruction of a blood vessel in the brain; stroke.

ARTHRITIS: Painful inflammation of a joint or joints of the body, usually producing heat and redness. The condition can be brought about by nerve impairment, increased or decreased function of the endocrine glands, or degeneration due to age.

ATARACTIC: A tranquilizing drug; of or having to do with tranquilizing drugs or their effects.

ATHEROSCLEROSIS: A thickening and loss of the elasticity in the inner walls of the arteries and accompanied by the deposition of atheromas or fatty nodules.

BIOLOGICAL ASSAY: A means of estimating the strength or potency of a drug by using some living organism or animal. The strength of the unknown sample is compared with a known or standard drug.

CALLUS: A mass of undifferentiated cells that develops over cuts or wounds on plants as at the ends of stem or leaf cuttings.

CANCER: Common term for a neoplasm, or a tumor, that is malignant. A large portion of human cancers may be caused by various chemicals, such as nitrites, some steroids, asbestos, smoking, radiation, viruses, etc.

CARCINOGEN: Any agent or substance that produces or causes cancer.

CARCINOMA: Any of several kinds of cancerous growths made up of epithelial cells.

CARDIOVASCULAR: Referring to the heart and the blood vessels as a unified body system.

CARMINATIVE: Having the power to relieve flatulence and colic.

CASTRATON: The removal of the testicles; gelding.

CEREBROVASCULAR: Referring to the brain and the blood vessels as a unified body system.

CHEMOTHERAPY: The prevention or treatment of infection by the systemic administration of chemical drugs.

CHOLESTEROL: A sterol, or fatty alcohol, found especially in animal fats, blood, nerve tissue, and bile and thought to be a factor in atherosclerosis.

CHOLINE: A viscuous liquid ptomaine, found in many animal and vegetable tissues: a vitamin of the B complex.

CHROMATOGRAPHY: A method of analysis in which the flow of the solvent or gas promotes the separation of substances by differential migration from a narrow inital zone in a porous sorptive medium. Four types generally employed are: column, paper, thin-layer, and gas.

COMPONENT: An element or ingredient; any of the main constituent parts.

CONSTITUENT: An essential part, component. The chemical entities contained in a crude drug.

CONSUMPTION: A disease that causes the body or part of the body to waste away; especially tuberculosis of the lungs.

CONVULSION: A violent, involuntary contraction or spasm of the muscles.

CRUDE DRUGS: Naturally occurring materials of animal, plant, and mineral origin that have not been chemically processed or purified.

DEBILITATING DISEASE: Any disease that causes a weakening of a patient.

DEBILITY: Weakness, feebleness, languor of body.

DEGENERATION: Deterioration of mentality; deterioration in structure or function of cells, tissues, or organs, as in disease or aging.

DEMULCENT: Medicine or ointment that soothes irritated or inflamed mucous membrane.

DEPRESSANT: A drug or medicine that lowers the rate of muscular, nervous activity.

DEPRESSION: An emotional state of dejection usually associated with manic-depressive psychosis.

DEPRESSOR: A nerve, stimulation of which by an agent, lowers arterial blood pressure by reflex vasodilation and by slowing the heart.

DIABETES: An inheritable, constitutional disease of unknown cause, characterized by the failure of the body tissues to oxidize carbohydrate at a normal rate. Its most important factor is a deficiency of insulin.

DIASTASE: An enzyme from malt that converts starch to maltose by hydrolysis.

DISPENSATORY: A book containing a systematic discussion of medicinal agents, including origin, preparation, description, uses and modes of action.

DNA (DESOXYRIBONUCLEIC ACID): A type of nucleic acid, found in animal and plant cells, occurring in the nuclei; it contains phosphoric acid, D-2-desoxyribose, adenine, guanine, cytosine, and thymine. The substance from normal cells appears to differ from that of cancer cells.

DOSAGE FORM: The physical state in which a drug or drugs is dispensed, such as tablets, capsules, or injectables, suitable for drug delivery to the patient.

DOSE: The amount of drug needed at a given time to produce a particular or clinically desired activity or effect.

DYSPEPSIA: Disturbed digestion; indigestion; impaired digestion.

EDEMA: Excessive accumulation of fluid in the tissue spaces; due to disturbance in the mechanisms of fluid exchange.

EEG (ELECTROENCEPHALOGRAM): A tracing showing the changes in electric potential produced by the brain.

ELEUTHEROSIDE: A biologically active saponin glycoside, isolated from the root of Siberian ginseng, having varied but similar, activities of ginseng glycosides.

ENDOCRINE GLANDS: Any of the ductless glands, such as the adrenals, the thyroid, the pituitary, whose secretions pass directly into the blood stream.

ENZYME: A catalyst of protein nature, which accelerates biological reactions but remains apparently unchanged itself, when the reaction is completed.

ERYTHROCYTE: A red blood corpuscle; it is a very small, circular disk with both faces concave, and contains hemoglobin, which carries oxygen to the body tissues.

ESTROGEN: Any of a group of female hormones. The estrogens cause the thickening of the lining of the uterus and vagina in the early phase of menstruation; responsible for female secondary sex characteristics. Estradiol, estrone, and estriol account for most of the estrogenic activity.

EXCIPIENT: An inert substance or substances used to give a pharmaceutical dosage form suitable for delivery.

EXPECTORANT: A remedy that promotes or modifies the amount of fluid or semifluid matter from the lungs and air passages expelled by coughing and spitting.

FATIGUE: Inability to perform reasonable and necessary physical and or mental activity. Fatigue may be associated with systemic disorders such as anemia, deficiency of nutrition, oxygen, addiction to drugs, endocrine gland disorders, or kidney disorders in which there is a large accumulation of waste products, or psychic disorders, etc. Excess fatigue causes exhaustion.

FLAVONOID: Any of the flavone derivatives, including citrin, hesperetin, hesperidin, rutin, quercetin, and quercitrin, which may reduce capillary fragility in certain cases.

GASTROENTERITIS: Inflammation of stomach and intestines.

GENIN: A term used to refer to the aglycone or nonsugar portion of glycosides in plants.

GINSENGENIN: The genin or aglycone of *Panax ginseng* extracted by alcohol.

GINSENOSIDE: Japanese term referring to a number of ginseng saponin glycosides isolated from the methanol extract of *Panax ginseng* root.

GLYCOSIDE: Substance that on hydrolysis yields one or more sugars and genin, or aglycone. The sugar portion is called glycone. The most important glycosides-containing plants are digitalis, rhubarb, aloe, glycyrrhiza, ginseng, etc.

GLYCOSURIA: The presence of sugar in the urine.

GONADOTROPIC: A substance (hormone) that is gonad-stimulating.

HEMATINIC: A blood tonic that increases the formation of hemoglobin and red blood cells.

HEMODYNAMICS: The study of how the physical properties of the blood and its circulation through the vessels affect blood flow and pressure.

HEMOGLOBIN: The red coloring matter of the red blood corpuscles, a protein yielding heme and globin on hydrolysis; it carries oxygen from the lungs to tissues and carbon dioxide from the tissue to the lungs.

HEMOLYTIC: Referring to the destruction of red blood cells and the escape of hemoglobin.

HERBAL: Referring to a plant used for medicinal purposes or for its odor or flavor.

HISTAMINE: An amine, produced by the decarboxylation of histidine and found in all organic matter; it is released by the tissues in allergic reaction, lowers the blood pressure by dilating blood vessels, stimulates gastric secretion, etc.

HISTAMINIC: Causing the stimulation of the visceral muscles, dilation of the capillaries, stimulation of the salivary, pancreatic, and gastric secretions.

HOMEOSTASIS: The maintenance of steady states in the organism by coordinated physiologic processes. Thus all organ systems are integrated by automatic adjustments to keep within narrow limits disturbances excited by the changes in the organism or in the surroundings of the organism.

HORMONE: Active principles secreted by endocrine glands: epinephrine, thyroxin, insulin, estradiol, testosterone, etc.

HYPERGLYCEMIA: Excess of sugar in the blood.

HYPERGLYCEMIC: Referring to the condition, hyperglycemia.

HYPERTENSION: Excessive tension, usually synonymous with high blood pressure.

HYPERTENSIVE: Referring to hypertension.

HYPNOTIC: A remedy that causes sleep; inducing sleep.

HYPOGLYCEMIA: The condition produced by a low level of sugar in the blood.

HYPOGLYCEMIC: Referring to the condition hypoglycemia.

HYPERTENSION: Excessive tension, usually synonymous with high blood pressure.

HYPERTENSIVE: Referring to hypertension.

HYPNOTIC: A remedy that causes sleep; inducing sleep.

HYPOGLYCEMIA: The condition produced by a low level of sugar in the blood.

HYPOGLYCEMIC: Referring to the condition hypoglycemia.

HYPOTENSION: Diminished or abnormally low tension, usually synonymous with low blood pressure.

HYPOTENSIVE: Referring to hypotension.

IMPOTENCE: Inability of the male to perform sexual intercourse. Impotence may result from physical causes such as structural abnormalities of the genital organs; decreased activity of the thyroid, pituitary, or sex glands; anemia, or other debilitating diseases; alcoholism; or may be psychological in origin.

INFLAMMATION: The reaction of the tissues to injury. The essential process, regardless of the causative agent, is characterized clinically by local heat, swelling, redness, and pain.

INSOMNIA: Sleeplessness; disturbed sleep; a prolonged condition of inability to sleep.

INTRAPERITONEAL: Within the peritoneum or peritoneal cavity.

IN VITRO: In glass; referring to a process or reation carried out in a culture dish, testtube, etc.

IN VIVO: In the living organism: used in contrast to *in vitro.*

KETOACIDOSIS: Acidosis accompanied by an increase in the blood of such ketones as β-hydroxybutyric, and acetoacetic acids.

LD_{50} (LETHAL DOSE 50): The dosage by which fifty percent of the experimental animals die.

LEUKEMIA: Any disease of the blood-forming organs, resulting in an abnormal increase in the production of leukocytes often accompanied by anemia and enlargement of the lymph nodes, spleen, and liver.

LEUKOCYTE: One of the colorless, more or less ameboid cells of the blood, having a nucleus and cytoplasm.

LEUKOCYTOSIS: Increase in the leukocyte count above the upper limits of normal.

LEUKOPENIA: A decrease below the normal number of leukocytes in the peripheral blood.

LONGEVITY: Term denoting the length or duration of the life used to indicate an unusually long life.

MALAISE: A general feeling of illness, lack of appetite, and decreased energy.

MAST CELLS: A cell containing large, easily dye-stained granules, found in connective and other body tissues.

MATERIA MEDICA: The division of pharmacology that treats the sources, descriptive, and preparations of substances used in medicine.

METABOLISM: Sum of all biochemical processes involved in life, two subcategories of metabolism are anabolsm, the building up of complex organic molecules from simpler precursors, and catabolism, the breakdown of complex substances into simpler molecules, often accompanied by the release of energy; metabolic reactions are usually catalyzed by enzymes.

MUSCARINIC: Stimulating the parasympathetic nerves and slowing of the heartbeat; increasing the secretions of the salivary.

NEPHRITIS: Inflammation of the kidney.

NEURASTHENIA: A group of symptoms ascribed to debility or exhaustion of the nerve centers; fatigability, lack of energy, various aches and pains, and disinclination to activity.

NEUROGENIC: Of nervous origin; stimulated by the nervous system.

NEUROSIS: A disorder of the psyche of psychic functions.

NORMALIZATION: Reduction to normal or standard state.

ONCOLOGY: The study or science of neoplastic growth (cancer).

ORGANISM: Any living entity having differentiated members with specialized functions that are interdependent, and that is so constituted as to form a unified whole capable of carrying on life processes.

PANAQUILIN: Group of nine ginseng saponin glycosides successfully isolated and identified from American ginseng root.

PANAXADIOL: A substance (genin) yielded from panaxosides after acid hydrolysis.

PANAXOSIDE: Soviet term referring to a number of ginseng saponin glycosides isolated from the methanol extracts of *Panax ginseng* roots.

PANAXATRIOL: A substance (genin) yielded from panaxosides after acid hydrolysis.

PAPAVARINLIKE: Having a local anesthetic or muscle-relaxing effect.

PARALYSIS: Partial or complete loss or temporary interruption, of a function, especially of voluntary motion or of sensation in some parts or all of the body.

PEN-TS'AO: The compendium dealing with crude drugs. The first *Pen-ts'ao* is called *Shen-nung Pen-ts'ao ching* formally published in the second century. The most complete *Pen-ts'ao* is *Pen-ts'ao Kang-mu* published by Li, Shih-chen in 1596.

pH: A chemical symbol used to express acidity and alkalinity in terms of the hydrogen ion concentration. The pH values may range from 0 to 14, numbers less than 7 indicating acidic, and numbers greater than 7, indicating basic.

PHARMACOGNOSY: The science dealing with the preparation, uses, and properties of crude drugs. In a broad sense, pharmacognosy embraces the knowledge of the history, distribution, cultivation, collection, selection, preparation, commerce, identification, evaluation, preservation, and use of drugs and other agents affecting the health of man and animals.

PHOSPHOLIPID: A type of lipid compound that is an ester of phosphoric acid and contains, in addition, one or two molecules of fatty acid, an alcohol, and a nitrogenous base, such as lecithin, cephalin, and sphingomyelin.

PHYTOSTEROL: Any of several steroid alcohols found in plants.

PLACEBO: A biologically inert substance, such as lactose, that is used as a sham drug. The placebo has no inherent pharmacological activity, but may produce a biologic response.

POLYURIA: Excessive urination, as in some diseases.

PRESSOR: Designating a nerve that, when stimulated, causes a rise in blood pressure; a substance capable of raising blood pressure.

PSYCHASTHENIA: A group of neuroses characterized by phobias, obsessions, undue anxiety, etc.

PSYCHOPHARMACOLOGY: The study of the actions of drugs on the mind.

PULSE: Alternate expansion and contraction of artery walls as heart action varies blood volume within the arteries. Usually, the pulse rate is determined by counting the pulsations per minute in the radial artery at the wrist. Various diseases may be indicated by changes in the rate, rhythm, and force of the pulse.

PULSOLOGY: The study and science of pulse.

PYRETIC: Of, causing, or characterized by fever.

REJUVENATION: A renewal of youth; a renewal of strength and vigor; specifically, a restoration of sexual vigor.

R_f VALUE: The ratio of the distance traveled on the plate or paper by the test substances to the distance traveled by the solvent front of the mobile phase, from the point of application of the test substance.

RHEUMATISM: A popular term of any of various painful conditions of the joints and muscles, characterized by inflammation, stiffness, etc., and including rheumatoid arthritis, bursitis, neuritis, etc.

RHEUMATOID ARTHRITIS: A chronic disease whose cause is unknown, characterized by inflammation, pain, and swelling of the joints accompanied by spasms in adjacent muscles and often leading to deformity in the joints.

RNA (RIBONUCLEIC ACID): Nucleic acid occurring in cell cytoplasma and the nucleolus, first isolated from plants, but later found also in animal cells, containing phosphoric acid, D-ribose, adenine, guanine, cytosine, and uracil.

SAPOGENIN: Term referring to the nonsugar portion of ginseng saponin glycosides.

SAPONIN: Saponins are characterized by forming colloidal solutions in water that foam upon shaking, have a bitter, acrid taste, and are irritating to the mucous membrane; hemolytic to blood cells.

SEDATIVE: Quieting function or activity.

SHOCK: The clinical manifestations of defective venous return to the heart with consequent reduction in cardiac output. It may be caused by inadequate pumping by the heart, by reduction of the blood volume due to dehydration, or to loss of blood or plasma, or by reduced blood pressure resulting from dilation of the blood vessels.

SIDE-EFFECT: Drug-induced symptoms that may be undesirable.

STIGMASTEROL: A sterol derived from the soybean.

STIMULANT: An agent that causes increased functional activity.

STOMACHIC: One of the class of substances that may stimulate the secretory activity of the stomach.

STRESS: Any stimulus or succession of stimuli or such magnitude as to tend to disrupt the homeostasis of the organism.

SYNERGISM: The response or action of one drug is enhanced by the other, synergism occurs. The term potentiation has been used for synergism.

SYNERGISTIC: Referring to synergism.

TLC (thin layer chromatography): Characterized by the application of dry, finely powdered absorbent in a thin, uniform layer to a glass plate. This plate is comparable to an open chromatographic column, and the separation of the components in the test material is based on absorption, partition, depending on the absorbents and the solvent used. Identification of an unknown component is made by comparing its R_f value with that of the known (standard) material.

TONIC: An agent or drug given to improve the normal tone of an organ, or of the patient generally.

TONIC EFFECT: Mentally or morally invigorating; stimulating.

TRYPANOSOMA: Slender, elongate organisms with a central nucleus, posterior blepharoplast, and an undulatory membrane, from which a free flagellum projects forward.

VITALITY: Mental or physical vigor; energy.

VOLATILE OILS: Essential oils that represent the odoriferous principles of plants: peppermint oil, clove oil, rose oil, etc.

INDEX OF NAMES

239

INDEX OF SUBJECTS